It's Just That Simple ...

Weight Loss, Workouts & Wellness
for the Overweight & Obese

Bruce A. Lea, M.A.

Book Information

It's Just That Simple ...
Weight Loss, Workouts & Wellness
for the Overweight & Obese

ISBN 978-1537272900

Printed by Createspace,
an Amazon.com Company

First Printing, 2016

Cover Art: GlinskajaOlga (istockphoto)

To my wonderful wife of many years …

who after reading this book for the very first time, said

"Wow, I thought you were just screwing around all this time …

this book is REALLY, REALLY GOOD!"

Hahahaha … what a glowing endorsement!

Thanks for being everything that you are.

Table of Contents

1.	**WORTH NOTING**	**7**
2.	**INTRODUCTION**	**9**
3.	**MY STORY**	**15**
4.	**WEIGHT LOSS**	**27**
4.1	The Diet and a Definition	29
4.2	The Diet and Goal Setting	30
4.3	The Diet and Its Theory	33
4.4	The Diet and the First Step	37
4.5	The Diet and Its Application	39
4.6	The Diet and Fiber Intake	45
4.7	What About Other Diets?	48
4.8	Beware the Low Carb Flu	51
5.	**WORKOUT (GENERAL INFO)**	**55**
5.1	Excuses, Excuses	58
5.2	When to Work Out	61
5.3	Where to Work Out	63
5.3.1	Working Out at Home	64
5.3.2	Working Out at a Gym	67
5.4	What to Wear	72
5.5	Aches and Pains	76
5.6	Remember the RICE	78
5.7	How to Work Out	81
5.8	The Stool of Fitness	85
6.	**WORKOUT (AEROBIC)**	**87**
6.1	Aerobic Info (General)	89
6.2	Aerobic Training … It Works	95
6.3	Start Your Aerobic Engine	100
7.	**WORKOUT (STRENGTH)**	**106**
7.1	Push and Pull	108
7.2	Language Requirement	110
7.3	Strength Training Methods	111
7.4	Beginning Your Strength Program	116
7.5	Basic Workout for Beginners	119
7.6	The Exercises	122
7.7	Circuit Training	134

7.8	Breathe In, Breathe Out	136
7.9	Personal Observations	137
	7.9.1 Perception	138
	7.9.2 Magazine Syndrome	139
	7.9.3 Everything Old is New Again	140
	7.9.4 Feeling Frustrated ... Functionally	141
8.	**WELLNESS**	**146**
8.1	Wellness Defined	146
8.2	Wellness Through the Ages	149
	8.2.1 Wellness in Antiquity	151
	8.2.2 Wellness 1400 CE – 1800 CE	155
	8.2.3 Wellness 1800 CE – 2000 CE	157
	8.2.4 Wellness 2000 CE – Present	165
8.3	The Wellness Pie	171
8.4	Emotional Wellness	173
8.5	Occupational Wellness	179
	8.5.1 What is Occupational Wellness?	179
	8.5.2 You and Your Occupation	181
8.6	Spiritual Wellness	187
	8.6.1 What Is Spiritual Wellness?	189
	8.6.2 Spiritual or Religious?	191
	8.6.3 Spiritual Wellness and Your Health	196
8.7	Intellectual Wellness	203
	8.7.1 How Can I Improve My Intellectual Wellness?	206
	8.7.2 When It Comes to Your Brain, Use Your Head	208
8.8	Social Wellness	213
	8.8.1 Origins of Social Wellness	213
	8.8.2 Social Wellness and Your Health	215
	8.8.3 So What Happened To Us?	219
	8.8.4 Maximize Your Social Wellness	225
8.9	Physical Wellness	231
	8.9.1 Physical Activity	234
	8.9.2 Proper Nutrition	237
	8.9.3 Effective Healthcare	239
	8.9.4 Oh, and One More Thing	242

9. CONCLUSION   247
10. REFERENCES   250

1.   WORTH NOTING

Two important tidbits on this page ... a medical disclaimer and a brief explanation of the book format. I know you can hardly wait to get to "the good stuff", but you can surely afford two minutes to read this information.

First, I have to put this in, so here it goes ... SEE A DOCTOR BEFORE YOU BEGIN THIS OR ANY DIETARY CHANGES OR WORKOUT REGIMEN. Whew, glad that's finished. Here is what you really need to pay attention to ... regular medical checkups are important to us all. To the overweight and obese among us, regular doctor visits are especially crucial. In my experience, a large percentage of really big people avoid the doctor completely. Quit sticking your head in the sand ... find yourself a primary care physician and go see them. All doctors aren't for all patients. If you don't like the first one, keep looking until you find one that you can connect with. You need to be able to establish a good rapport with your medical team. Don't be afraid or ashamed to seek medical advice. The function of physicians is to help you, so go see one.

Second, the book is written in a pretty straightforward, fairly easy to follow format, with the chapters consisting of a variety of relevant information. At various places throughout each chapter, you may find a "*Personally...*" section where I relate an experience of mine (or of someone I know) to the info in the chapter.

I look forward to hearing your stories as you journey to wellness. If you have questions, comments, or personal stories to share, feel free to contact me at:

pathway4wellness@gmail.com

2   INTRODUCTION

Welcome to *"It's Just That Simple..."* Lots of people want to write a book ... this is mine. This particular project actually began as more of a text book style venture ... but as I would read it, it became apparent that a text book format wouldn't work. Not that I'm not a magnificent writer, with great command of the English language ... because I am (hahaha) ... but I realized that the answer to being a "better you" is so simple that I would only run the risk of boring the reader. The result of the change in direction is the much more informal product you are reading. So why buy this book and read it? Simply put, to regain control of your body and in doing so, reduce weight, strengthen your body, and improve your health and overall wellness ... basically so you'll feel much better about yourself.

So you want to lose weight and become healthier, huh? I promise this plan is as simple as it can be ... but not always easy to do. That's right ... SIMPLE, BUT NOT EASY. Deal with it. So often today, people want something that is based on masses of longitudinal studies and reams of research, and at the same time is really easy to accomplish. They want a pill, a shot, something to sprinkle ... in other words, they want anything besides getting out of their comfort zone. If you haven't figured it out by now, the truth is that a really easy path doesn't exist. Suck it up, buttercup.

Next, if you haven't thrown the book down yet, I must ask you to do something before we proceed. Do a quick self examination, and answer this question as honestly as possible ... *are you considered overweight ... or obese ... or even morbidly obese*? If so, then please read this book. If you need to lose ten pounds or less to achieve the body beautiful, this book probably isn't for you. Unless you are buying it for someone else, just put the book down and walk away slowly. While I sincerely appreciate the fact that you chose to occupy your most valuable resource (your time) by studying my work, I feel obligated to tell you that this book is designed for the fatties among us.

The *fatties*, huh? Let's face it, you know who you are. You are the person who wonders how the picture of the fatso got on your driver's license. Or the guy who hates to go anywhere requiring a tie, because buttoning a shirt around your neck is a chore ... maybe even a two person job. Maybe you are the gal who is the "big girl" ... you know, the one who is "sweet" with the "really pretty face" and the "great personality." You avoid airplane travel because you can't fit in the seats ... or would need to buy two seats ... or use a seat belt extender at the very least. Speaking of seat size, you don't really consider going to shows, plays, or movies because sitting comfortably (or even sitting at all) becomes an issue. When you wear your clothes, you often feel like a stuffed sausage. Many of you avoid having your picture taken. Any of this sound familiar?

How about some of these wonderfully flattering terms ... tubby, corn fed, pudgy, portly, bubble butt, muffin top, stout, thick, big un, fleshy, flabby, heavy set, beefy, round, lard butt, rotund, plump, roly-poly, etc. Be honest with yourself ... are you tired of being classified with this group of adjectives? If so, understand that I wrote this book for you.

I want to re-emphasize that this book was targeted at you guys and gals who are considered overweight or obese. It cannot be denied that carrying lots of extra weight is terribly *unhealthy*, is *not attractive* in societal terms, is *detrimental* to overall mental and physical health, and results in *self esteem issues*. The inescapable fact is that obese people are unhealthier, have a lower quality of life, and will die earlier. The most interesting part about what you just read is that ... obese people know all of this already.

Before I get swamped with letters from all the hefties out there who tell me that they are "happy being who they are", "comfortable with themselves", etc., I will tell you now that I am going to call BULL! While your mantra of becoming *one with your inner self* may sound good, I don't buy it for a second. There isn't one of you who can honestly say that you wouldn't prefer to lose 50, 100, 200 pounds or more. I assure you that if you follow the plan in this book, you could still be "who you are", only without carrying around the extra flab.

As I previously stated, this book outlines a wellness plan that is simple, but not always easy. There is no argument that habitual behavior like overeating is often terribly hard to overcome. And there is no doubt that overeating is an addiction

11

... a very powerful and very insidious obsession. So what is wrong with plump folks ... why can't they just slow down their eating? It's possible they would if they had the right tools to make it happen. Other addictions are the same ... for instance, there is not a smoker on the face of the earth who doesn't know that their habit is expensive, dirty, and unhealthy. I say this because I know that they would quit if they could ... but they can't. My daughter is a respiratory therapist, and as part of her job, she is required to take care of those who have breathing problems. Many of her patients are smokers, and she says that almost all of her patients plead with her to never start smoking ... they say they don't want anyone to end up in the same situation as them. Are all these people dumb, hopeless losers? Not a chance. I submit that they are a just cross-section of folks who have tried and failed because they have not found the right combination yet.

Along those same lines, fat folks know that being heavy is unhealthy, unsightly, and expensive in any number of ways. Like smokers, they too would beat their habit, drop the extra flab, and become lean and mean ... if they could. It is my experience that with the proper tools in their tool box, they too can overcome their devious addiction. I hope this book offers them the keys to crack the code to wellness.

So am I some sort of genius? Hardly. But I have been morbidly obese. I understand the personal struggles with diet, activity, and other aspects of obesity. Having lost a LOT of weight, I can tell you that I look a lot better, I am medically healthier, and most importantly, I feel a lot better. I want other overweight folks to have the opportunity to feel as good as I do. You deserve it ... the chance to feel better, both physically and mentally. To that end, this book was written to give the overweight and obese a fighting chance. If you want to take control of your life forever, read this book and follow the plan. Note the emphasis here on *you taking control of your life*. You will be amazed at how simple it really is ... not always easy, but excruciatingly simple ... hence, the title of the book. On the other hand, if you want to spend the rest of your life being overweight and "wishing I could", then keep doing what you're doing. As famed physicist Albert Einstein said, insanity can be defined as *doing the same thing over and over again and expecting different results.* Is this you?

Don't wait...*Carpe Diem...Seize the Day.*

Personally...

Okay, here is a scoop … please don't tell anyone, but just between us, I always admired workout guru Richard Simmons. No, it wasn't his wacky hair I admired … or the shiny little short shorts. No, what I appreciated was the fact that Simmons had been really fat, and had taken measures to reduce his weight and keep it off. In short, he had *been there, done that.* He created his "Deal a Meal" eating plan and coupled that with his "Sweatin to the Oldies" videos to assist folks in their journey to a healthier life. The thing that gave him the biggest buy-in was probably that he always used a lot of BIG PEOPLE in his videos … they were regular men and women … who could easily be your neighbors or family members … out there working hard to drop some poundage. I'm certain that is why he struck such a chord with so many people. Now contrast this with countless supermodels who will tell you about their eating habits and their workout plans, and how you should eat and exercise just like they do … yet who also are the same ones who binge and purge and undergo months of therapy if their weight zooms from 102 to 104! PLEASE!

3   MY STORY

Since you are reading this book, I can assume that you need to lose weight yourself, or know someone who does. This book contains a proven method to regain control of your life through a sustainable eating plan and the addition of movement and exercise, as well as information that will help you gain a balance in your life.

Unlike many others, I can relate to obese folks, since I have struggled against the food addiction for years. In fact, like any addiction, I will ALWAYS have to be mindful of what I take in. Even though I will need to be perpetually on guard, my perception is that I have complete control of myself, and want you to feel the same way. Along those lines, I feel it is important to give you a brief history of ... me! While everyone's story is a little different, I'm sure a lot of my past will ring true with many of you too.

I was always a "big" kid growing up. Growing up in the 1960s, I was pretty active. Of course, ALL kids were active then. After all, there were no video games, computers, smart phones ... you get the picture. Even television wasn't that much of a vice, since the programming was in black and white, and all stations went off the air no later than 11:00 p.m. In fact, a television station sign off was generally accomplished by playing the national anthem (which would certainly not be politically correct today, since it would undoubtedly offend one group or another!). In addition, most stations would say something like "It's 11:00 ... parents, do you know where your children are?" I wonder how many parents could answer that today? I still recall the wonder of watching shows such as Disney and Bonanza on our new *color* television set ... ah, sorry about the trip down memory lane ... I'll get back on track. So, even with all the bike riding, sports playing, and time spent outside, I was still a "big kid." I recall shopping for pants with my mom and always having to go to the "husky" section ... ugh. So, in retrospect I even started out on the wrong track.

As a child growing up in the South, I was exposed to lots of delicious food, primarily prepared at home. We ate quite a few vegetables and fruits, including greens, peas, beans, tomatoes, strawberries, watermelon, etc. That was the good news. On the flip side, as a normal southern family, a lot of our food choices came from one particular food group ... that would be the *Fried Food* group! God bless Southerners, they learned early on that you could roll almost anything in flour and fry it, and it would be delicious. While I had friends who were picky eaters, that didn't apply to me ... I ate EVERYTHING! I can still recall a typical meal at most any Southern home ... it might be something like fried chicken, rice with tomato gravy, lima beans, and some collard greens along with fresh biscuits. This would be followed by a big piece of pound cake which was fresh from the oven, which wasn't complete until it was smeared with butter, all washed down with copious amounts of iced tea ... sweet of course! There was also bread at every meal, whether it was the previously mentioned homemade biscuits, or cornbread, or that amazing health food, Wonder Bread. I recall the Wonder Bread slogan was "*Helps build strong bodies 12 ways.*" Really? And exactly what ... never mind, I'll let that go. Anyway ... in addition to all the other goodies, there was also a never ending supply of mashed potatoes, chicken and dumplings, homemade desserts, jellies & jams, etc.

I kept a handle on my weight though high school ... always a little big, but not out of control. After I graduated, I started attending community college during the mornings, heading off to work at a gas station every evening plus one day on the weekend. This schedule enabled me to have just enough time between school and work to hit a fast food drive-through for a quick meal. Then again at night, the diet might also be comprised of fast food, as well as beer, chips, etc. There is a common term that describes many college freshmen who put on weight ... it is called the *Freshman Fifteen*. Always an overachiever, I must have put on the *Freshman Fifty*! I graduated from the community college, and began taking classes at a nearby university, all the while maintaining my ever expanding body with garbage food.

About this time, I met a wonderful girl, and we started dating. Thankfully for me, approximately a year later she consented to become my wife (and lucky for me, at the time of writing this book we recently celebrated our 38th wedding anniversary). She was from a wonderful Italian family, and with apologies to Chef Boyardee, I was soon introduced to REAL Italian food. The meatballs, sausage, pasta, bread, meats, and cheeses were all new to me, and they were great! As a result of my affinity for the cuisine, my belly continued to expand.   Life continued to roll along, including the addition of two children and the loads of time that they required. I was working a job with rotating shifts, coaching sports teams, and having returned to college, I was attending classes as well. More fast food between ball fields, wrestling meets, and the college campus ...

Like many folks, I didn't really "see" my weight gain, but rather noticed it in my clothes. My clothes would always be tight and ill fitting. JC Penney became my sole clothing provider since they had a "Big and Tall" section. I marked my continued increasing girth by my clothing selections ... first there was XXL, then XXXL, and so on. Along the way, I tried a few half hearted attempts to curb my eating, but they weren't very successful, so not much changed.

Shortly after my kids had graduated from high school, I had to go to the doctor for some reason (I think it was exercise induced tendonitis in my elbow ... at least I was still working out a little!). Now, up to that time I might see a doctor every 5 or 6 years. Looking back, I may have subconsciously been afraid to go to the doctor, since he might be the bearer of bad news, but I'm certainly no psychologist, so who knows. The doc treated me for

18

my malady, and mentioned that my blood pressure was pretty high. I knew that my blood pressure had been slowly creeping up over the past decade (of course this is why they call it the *silent killer*), but I had put it out of my mind. So, the doc suggested that I return to him for a full physical, and I scheduled one ... although I felt I was still in pretty good shape. Of course, as part of the process, before the physical I went to the local lab and "donated" 4 or 5 vials of my blood for analysis. So by the time I arrived at my appointment, he had all of my information in his hot hands.

At the physical, the doc was not quite as impressed with my fitness level as I was. My weight was so high that I could barely weigh on the balance beam scale that was in his office. In addition, my blood pressure and cholesterol were both pretty high. This was especially disturbing to me, since although some of my family members were known to have blood pressure problems, not one of them was afflicted with cholesterol issues. Eye opener! To combat this, I was given a medication to reduce blood pressure, and I promised the doctor that I would adjust my food intake to address the cholesterol ... if that didn't work, I would consider medication for that as well.

This was quite a slap in the face. I became really angry with myself, asking what the hell was wrong with me. I decided to do some self-examination, and swore to determine what the problem was. I knew that my workouts had never really stopped throughout the years, although they had become sporadic. I felt confident that going forward, I could design and implement a successful workout program. However, I also knew deep down that my primary issues were with my diet.

So what were the main problems? After quite a bit of introspection, and *being honest with myself*, I soon realized that my issue was twofold. First, the quantity of food that I took in was much too large. Second, and most important for my future, I found that I ate too much from the carbohydrate group. In fact, I was addicted to carbohydrates. Make no mistake, it is an addiction as powerful as any. I could make a sandwich out of anything. I felt the need to add rice or potatoes to every meal. I ate big plates of pasta several times a week (loved me some Italian food). Even many of the foods I thought were okay (for instance lima beans, baked potatoes and most fruits) were FULL of carbohydrates.

Following the theory that it is often better to be lucky than good, I was fortunate that the Atkins diet was all the rage about that time. Of course, Dr. Atkins basically said that carbohydrates are bad and fats are good (please no emails from all you Atkins groupies ... I know it was more in-depth than that). I got the books, and after reading them, felt that they made pretty good sense. I had some of the same questions that others had, like how can I eat a pound of bacon and lose weight while still being healthy? Regardless, I decided that it might be just the thing to combat my addiction. It worked, and I lost 30 pounds in a fairly short time. However, as so often happens, I was not ready to stay on the diet long term, and I did not alter my workouts either. As a result, I slowly put most of the weight back on, and returned to still more unhealthy eating.

Having had some weight loss success by reducing my carbohydrate intake, I would later read with interest *The South Beach Diet* book by Dr. Agatston. It struck a chord deep inside me. It all made sense ... the proverbial light bulb came on. He didn't just dismiss all carbohydrates; rather, he broke them into good carbohydrates and bad carbohydrates. He did the same thing with fats, separating them into good and bad categories. For some reason, this really stuck with me. One thing I questioned (and still do) is the ability of this eating plan to help lose belly fat first ... I am certainly not a doctor, but I can't believe my body knows enough to lose belly fat any faster than fat from other body parts ... sorry to wander. Anyway, as I dove into this new eating plan, I immediately noticed that something was missing ... the feeling of being hungry! I was so used to equating a diet with being hungry, that I was shocked. The days of celery sticks and the like were gone. I was eating things I loved, such as turkey, chicken, ham, beef, salads, nuts, cheese, etc., and at the same time I wasn't hungry! Obviously, this plan was for me. I lost 75 pounds in the first 10 months, and I felt great. My energy level was higher than I could remember it being in years, and my blood pressure dropped about 35 points off of the "top number" and 20 off the "bottom number." As for my cholesterol, in the first six months it fell over 50 points. My doctor was really impressed, and actually was able to reduce my dosage of blood pressure medication. Quite frankly, I couldn't really believe it myself. I had found a way to eat that allowed me to ingest food that I liked, which had the byproduct of being dense enough to take a longer time for the body to process it, hence delaying hunger. At this particular stage, I hadn't done enough research to understand that the benefits of reduced carbohydrate eating included keeping your blood sugar in check as well, which not only paid dividends for weight loss, but also in a myriad of other ways. I'll discuss this more in Chapter 4, but suffice to say that carbohydrate reduction has long ranging positive effects on your body.

Back to my progress. I continued following this general path, and over the next few years, would slowly lose another 30 pounds. For several years, my weight floated between a net loss of 100 and 105 pounds. At this time, it had been about six years since I had begun the reduced carbohydrate plan from the South Beach series ... and I felt great. My workouts had been refined and I was actually firming up and increasing strength while at the same time dropping pounds.

While scanning the internet one day for low carbohydrate recipes, I stumbled across a few blogs that mentioned *The Protein Power Lifeplan* books by Dr. Michael & Mary Eads. They too advocated reduced carbohydrate eating, but with a slight twist.

They prefer to look at *net* carbohydrates, which is the total number of carbohydrates in any serving of food <u>MINUS</u> the fiber count in the same serving. Although the books did contain a lot of valuable medical info for the reader, to me the plan can be summarized by the suggestion that you eat anything, as long as your net carbohydrates stay under 30 per day. I know, it sounds too simple, but trust me.

Before we go further, I have to interject a pet peeve of mine here. Not sure it's the best place for it, but it's on my mind. I have probably heard most every excuse for not dieting, and more specifically, for not following a reduced carbohydrate plan. I will address many of these as we go through the book, but I can assure you of this ... when people start talking to me about changing their eating, I can generally tell within three minutes whether they are ready to follow my plan or not. They will spend time telling me why they can't follow it, which draws the same comment from me ... *you aren't ready to lose weight and change your life yet. When you feel you're really ready, get back with me and we can have a serious discussion.* One great example is the excuse that they don't want to have to look at numbers every time they want to eat something. My response? *You aren't ready for this diet. If you don't want to spend less than 10 minutes a day to find your total and net carbohydrates, then you obviously aren't serious about losing weight.* Ummm ... you may be able to tell that excuses drive me crazy ... especially poor excuses. So if you think you may want to give this plan a "try", I refer you to a world famous and well known philosopher ... *Yoda* from *Star Wars* ... who said, "Try not. Do ... or do not. There is no try." Ahem ... let's move on!

While monitoring your food intake by following net carbohydrates will result in weight loss, it also has the corollary benefit of raising your awareness about the amount of fiber intake each day. Since you are always subtracting the grams of fiber from the total carbohydrate count, you constantly have a running total of your fiber ingestion. Most folks are supposed to have in the neighborhood of 30 grams of fiber a day, but I submit that few people have the vaguest idea of how much they eat. We will hit this in more depth later, but just know that it is VERY important to eat a lot of fiber daily.

So, after adjusting my eating to stay under 30 net carbohydrates per day, my weight began to fall again ... this combination has proven to be even more successful. Note that for me, that success translates into around 120-125 pounds of blubber that I am not carrying around anymore. For further illustration, at the time I was reading the Protein Power books, a wonderful friend of mine finally reached her "moment of truth." She has a job that can be stressful, and along with bad eating habits, had allowed her weight to creep to its highest level ever. In addition, she was experiencing increasing health issues. So, she began following the Protein Power plan of staying below 30 net carbohydrates. In one year, she has lost over 40 pounds, and has been able to reduce her blood pressure medicine. Again, this stuff works.

Along with the weight loss, I became interested in achieving a balance in life. I continued to manipulate my workout composition, took up several new hobbies, read a variety of books on an assortment of subjects, joined a fraternal organization, created my own company, and many other things. While I didn't exactly know it at the time, I had taken steps to increase my *wellness*. While we will go much, much deeper into the topic of wellness later in this book, suffice to know that wellness depends on a balance of the body, mind, and spirit to function properly.

So to reiterate, I want to reach the people that most need this information ... the overweight and obese folks. If you need to lose weight ... and I mean really lose weight ... you owe it to yourself to follow the plan that I have outlined for you in this book. You will feel better, both inside and out. Your overall wellness will increase. I assure you this ain't some infomercial. This is real life ... mine. Make it happen for you too. You're worth it.

Personally...

I feel that I have extremely good control of my diet, especially when it comes to carbohydrates. However, I also know that it will be a lifetime struggle. How do I know? Because I still get urges for some of my old comfort food. For instance, if I am at a restaurant and a big plate of fresh, extra crispy french fries passes by, I have to fight the urge to tackle the server! I went for 7 years without one single french fry. Now that I have control of my habits, a few times a year I will indulge in a small order of fries just for fun. In fact, once a year around my birthday, I go out to a restaurant and order a double burger and fries ... and I eat every single bite, crumb, and morsel! I polish off the burger, the bun, the fries, and will even slop the fries in copious amounts of catsup. After that, I feel bloated, sluggish and generally horrible as the result of my body trying to process this load of junk I just stuffed in. This serves as my annual reminder that the old adage "garbage in, garbage out" is painfully true. It also serves to help me to avoid further dumb choices ... well, at least until my next birthday!

4   WEIGHT LOSS

"Knowing is not enough; we must apply.
Willing is not enough; we must do."
Johann von Goethe (German writer, statesman)

If you are reading this book, it would probably be safe to assume you are interested in weight loss. As you are already aware, you don't feel good while carrying too much weight around ... unhealthy, looks, etc. The entire purpose of this book is to enable those very readers like you to use weight loss, workouts, and wellness to achieve a life balance.

One important thing to understand is that there are a myriad of reasons people eat too much food, and those types of eating patterns never solve problems. Losing weight is vital for many. In contrast, don't expect weight loss to be a magic potion for all of life's ills either. As our pal and television host Phillip McGraw (better known as Dr. Phil) says, "At your goal weight or not, you still have to live with yourself and deal with your problems. You will still have the same husband, the same job, the same kids, and the same life. Losing weight is not a cure for life" (McGraw 2003). Well said, Doc.

All things considered, there is no doubt that eating the wrong amount and types of food causes you to be obese. In this section we will provide you the tools needed to gain control of your food intake. Since we know that food intake is our problem, it is imperative that we take heed of the quote above by von

Goethe ... we have the knowledge, and need to be willing to apply that knowledge. Each person reading this book has to gain mastery over their own food intake. The eating plan described here is the cornerstone of the program that will allow you to do that ... it helps you to break from past habits. I estimate that diet is approximately sixty percent of getting control of your body again (your workout will comprise the other forty percent). It should be apparent that if you can restructure your eating plan, you will be well on the road to recovering your body ... and your life. Follow this plan for any and all reasons that you can imagine ... but more than anything, follow it for yourself.

The Diet and a Definition

Finally … we're ready to dive into the eating plan for weight loss. Before we go any further, we need to define the word *diet*. For most people, the word "diet" is considered a "four letter word" … you know, one of the words that you should mention to the priest during confession, or ones that would get your mouth washed out with soap when you were younger! The bad rap that diets have gotten is because they represent a major change for people … a symbol of an uncomfortable eating plan … something sinister. It is probably a good idea to refer to Merriam-Webster's online dictionary that says a diet is:

a: food and drink regularly provided or consumed

b: habitual nourishment

c: a regimen of eating and drinking sparingly so as to reduce one's weight

You can see that the last definition is the one people typically relate to the word. For our purposes during the remainder of this book, when the term "diet" comes up, please note that it can be thought of as *food and drink regularly provided or consumed,* or as *habitual nourishment.* It is not to be considered as a term regarding a weight loss regimen. It shouldn't have a negative stigma attached to it … a helpful diet ain't all that bad!

The Diet and Goal Setting

I hear it all the time .... "I need to lose about fifteen pounds" ... or "If I could lose ten more pounds I could fit into that dress". Quite frankly, having been really heavy, that thought process makes me crazy! So, all you heavy folks, for maybe the first time in your life I am going to give you some sage advice ... don't obsess over the numbers on the bathroom scale! In my experience, all that does is to set you up for failure.

You're probably excited about an author telling you to forget about getting on a scale ... nice try. It's still necessary to weigh yourself occasionally to see how you are progressing. Please don't weigh yourself every day ... or even several times a day ... and expect it to mean anything. Genuine weight loss is accomplished over weeks and months, not minutes! I suggest that you weigh yourself no more than one day a week, and at the same time of day each time. Oh, and as for scales, there are endless varieties and styles. I recommend the balance beam style scale ... more expensive, but they are much more reliable.

I can hear you now, all asking "But how can knowing what you weigh be a bad thing?" It really isn't, provided you don't believe it to be the only variable that you need to monitor. Obviously, you have to know a baseline number to determine how you are progressing with your plan. However ... let's say for example that you set a goal of losing 60 pounds in a year. You follow the plan, you feel like you did really well, but you only lose

45 pounds. Is that a failure? I submit to you that losing 45 pounds is a tremendous achievement, particularly in a year. But you didn't reach your goal ... are you a loser? After all, your goal was 60. Or the flip side ... how about if you lose the 60 pounds ... now what? Do you stop? Do you set yet another goal for the next year? How good does that make your first goal? My message here is that you need to change your way of thinking ... you need to forget about chasing some particular number on a scale, but instead concentrate on changing your way of eating for life.

Also, based on body types and a lot of other things, *pounds* are not always the best indicator of fitness / wellness. There are folks at 180 pounds who are extremely out of whack physically, and 240 pounders who aren't too shabby. Work with your health care team to get control of all your risk factors.

Another questionable indicator is the body's *BMI* (Body Mass Index). BMI is commonly used to determine if someone is overweight … or obese … or morbidly obese. As an equation, BMI is a person's body mass divided by the square of their height. I know ... please Bruce, no calculations! Okay, how about ... *BMI is a number representing how thick or thin a person is*. Better? If BMI is used as one of many tools to determine relative fitness, it would be fine. However, BMI doesn't factor in the size of the body's frame, so a small framed person may be thicker and fatter but with a BMI in the normal range. Flipping that around, it is also possible that a person with a larger more muscular frame may

31

have a low body fat reading, but their BMI says they are overweight or worse. So like all tools, BMI should be used not as a stand-alone measure, but rather as part of a more comprehensive diagnostic battery.

As for goals, you may not believe this, but I can honestly say that when I started my new eating style almost twelve years ago, I never had a goal weight in mind. NEVER. I knew that I was too heavy, and that I had to make my weight go down. I never had a goal weight then ... and I don't have one today. If I eat cleanly and continue to work out regularly, my body will slowly make the changes it needs to as it adapts (and it does). Don't obsess over the reading on your scale ... even when the weight may not be falling off of you, your improved eating habits result in the cleaning of your body on the inside, which is a valuable result as well. This all goes back to regarding this way of living as a plan for life, not just a temporary change.

The Diet and Its Theory

All right, let's get to it. The diet that has worked for me (and will work for you) is based on restricting your carbohydrate intake. As I have noted in other parts of this book, I have been influenced in varying ways by the reduced carbohydrate standards of our day, including Atkins, South Beach, and Protein Power. These programs all agree that to lose weight and clean the insides, you must limit your carbohydrate intake. They each have a slightly different approach, and I urge you to become well informed by reading these and other books, blogs, and available research on the topic. But, it basically boils down to reduction of carbohydrate intake. So how does reducing carbohydrates, while essentially forgetting about calories and fats, help you lose weight and increase your wellness? To address this question, it is probably best to review how carbohydrates work in your body. Relax, it's okay to learn something!

Like any engine, the body needs fuel to operate. In the average person, carbohydrates are the fuel. When you eat carbohydrates, your body recognizes the addition of these sugars and reacts by sending insulin into the blood. Your insulin directs the cells to use the sugar in the blood for fuel, and tells the fat cells not to worry, but to just stand by … they won't be needed because there are plenty of available carbohydrates to burn. The problem is that the body control mechanisms aren't all that precise. When you ingest carbohydrates, the blood glucose levels start to rise, and the body gets nervous. It shoots out insulin in large quantities to offset the anticipated sugar rush. So, although the insulin has done its job, the body doesn't know it yet. It will generally take out more sugar than it needs to ... which leads to you being hungry ... more specifically, craving more sweets. Note that in this context, "sweets" does not necessarily refer to a piece of cake, but can mean anything which is high in carbohydrates that the body can treat just like sugar. So, you tend to eat more carbohydrates to counter this craving, which has the effect of raising your blood glucose level up quickly. And what happens then? The body sees the high levels, dumps insulin, and the cycle continues. Therefore, eating carbohydrates creates peaks and valleys in your glucose levels, resulting in the need for insulin. While the body constantly struggles to find a happy medium for your glucose level, it actually protects the fat cells from being burned as fuel because it has plenty of sugar to use. These fat cells don't magically disappear ... they are stored in your body.

How can a reduced carbohydrate diet counter this? By reducing your carbohydrate intake, you moderate the yo-yo effect that exists in both the glucose levels and the amount of insulin released to counteract them. This reduces your food cravings ... in short, you aren't hungry any more. A bonus is that since the body still needs fuel to operate ... and you have drastically reduced the old fuel (carbs) ... it begins to burn fat for fuel, whether it is the fat

34

you just ate or your stored fat. Makes sense, huh? As a side note, the fact that your insulin levels stay moderated makes this a great eating plan for those who are prone to diabetes, since blood sugar stays fairly level.

Next, let me cause a real poop storm by stating ... the body needs fat, the body needs protein, but the body really doesn't need a lot of carbohydrates. At this point, I can hear all the dieticians leaping out of their chairs and screaming ... however, it's a true statement. Carbohydrates can be reduced drastically without any noticeable effect. This most likely comes from some genetic wiring we developed through our evolution. Face it, meat has been around a LONG time. We've all read about the ancestors killing big animals like a mastodon and using all the meat, hide, and tusks. While they also ate nuts, berries, and leaves, meat was a staple. It is important to realize that most carbohydrates are the result of something being grown and/or processed. Since organized agriculture is a fairly recent event in our past, it is apparent that humans ate meat long before the onset of carbohydrates.

I can tell you from personal experience that one of the main things I know about this way of eating is that I am never hungry. I'll tell you honestly that if I'm hungry, it's my own fault. Anyone I have ever encountered that has success with reduced carbohydrate eating will give the lack of hunger as one of the biggest reasons for the success. Reduced carbohydrate eating has been referred to as *self limiting* … that is, by eating proteins and fats you become full and satisfied without packing in lots of food. This food is also typically more dense, requiring the body to process it more completely; in other words, the residence time in the body is longer, helping to offset the hungry, empty feeling. This eating style results in a different type of full … you become satiated, but not bloated.

The Diet and the First Step

So, you bought this great book, and you are fired up and ready to change your future. Are you ready to head to the store and buy all of this low carbohydrate stuff to eat? Sounds good, but before you go to the store, you should probably make one quick stop first. Without a doubt, your first step to beginning and following this diet is to ... GO SEE YOUR DOCTOR! Please don't get aggravated with my preaching about doctors ... I promise that the American Medical Association does not have me on retainer! I just know personally about the wellness advantages to creating a relationship with a primary care physician. If you don't have one, get one. You can look in the mirror to see what you look like on the outside, but you have no idea what is happening on the inside. I beg with you, I plead with you, I beseech you ... GO SEE A DOCTOR! Many folks, particularly those who are really heavy, avoid doctors at all costs. Embarrassment, fear, who knows why. Get a physical for God's sake. I assure you they have seen big folks before. What the hell, even after losing over 120 pounds I sure ain't gonna be wearing a Speedo to the beach ... but I AM going to my doctor regularly! I know this disclaimer will give all lawyers everywhere a warm fuzzy feeling, but I mention it for your own well being.

In fact, while you are at the doctors' office, tell the doc that you want to lose weight by following the plan laid out in this book. Unless the doc has valid reasons for you not to, you will eat a reduced carbohydrate diet, increase your workouts / activity levels, and address any areas that are out of balance in your life to achieve some level of wellness. I predict your medical pro will be excited that you are ready to make changes. Oh, and please feel free to tell them to buy a few hundred copies of this book for their other patients too!

The Diet and Its Application

Okay, if you can count backwards from thirty to zero, you have the skill sets needed to handle this diet. No, really. If you can maintain an intake of less than thirty net carbohydrates a day, you will lose weight. What is a net carbohydrate? Think of your paycheck ... the gross pay is what you earned, while the net pay is what is left over after everything has been removed. Net carbohydrates are the same ... they are determined by taking the *Total Carbohydrates* in a serving of food, and then subtracting the *Total Fiber* and any *Sugar Alcohols* in the serving, resulting in your *Net carbohydrates*. This is the *whole basis of your eating plan for the rest of your life*, so here it is in bold print:

Total Carbohydrates - Total Fiber - Sugar Alcohols = Net Carbohydrates

In fact, since it appears everyone but me has a tattoo now, you may even want to hustle off to your local body art specialist and have this equation imprinted on some part of your body so that you can have it with you at all times for quick reference. And no, please don't feel the need to send me pictures of your new ink. Not too hard so far, huh? How about a few examples:

Ahhh...time for breakfast. Put some olive oil or butter (not margarine) in a pan and scramble a couple of eggs, throw in some bell peppers, some onion, and top it with some shredded cheese.

To give it a little Southwestern flavor, spread on about 2 tbsp of your favorite salsa before you eat. You choose to wash it all down with a couple of cups of coffee. The "carb cost" of this is shown in Table 4.1 below:

FOOD	SERVING SIZE	TOTAL CARBS	TOTAL FIBER	NET CARBS
Butter	3 tbsp	0	0	0
Egg	2 large	≈ 2	0	≈ 2
Bell Pepper	1/3 cup	≈ 2	≈ 1	≈ 1
Onion	1 tbsp	1	< 1	1
Cheddar Cheese	½ cup	< 1	0	< 1
Salsa	2 tbsp	2	0	2
Coffee	2 cups	0	0	0
Artificial Sweetener	2 packets	0	0	0
TOTALS		≈ 7	≈ 1	≈ 6

Table 4.1

You want a ham sandwich for lunch. You pull out the ham, lettuce, tomato, mayo, and mustard from the refrigerator. Now you get two pieces of white bread … NOOOOO! Two slices of average white bread will contain 28 grams of carbohydrates, with no fiber. That is almost your entire day's allocation of carbohydrates. Instead, you go into the pantry and retrieve 2 pieces of some low carbohydrate multi-grain bread you found at the local health food store. Much better. It has 10 carbohydrates per slice, but also has 8 grams of fiber per slice, which yields only 2 net carbohydrates per slice. Not only is it low in net carbohydrates, but it also gives you 16 grams of fiber, about half of your daily requirement. Now you can construct your

sandwich. The lunch results:

FOOD	SERVING SIZE	TOTAL CARBS	TOTAL FIBER	NET CARBS
Ham	3 slices	< 1	< 1	< 1
Mayonnaise (real)	3 tbsp	0	0	0
Yellow Mustard	1 tsp	0	0	0
Lettuce	2 leaves	0	0	0
Tomato	1 slice	<	< 1	< 1
Low Carb Bread	2 slices	20	16	4
TOTALS		≈ 20	≈ 16	≈ 4

Table 4.2

You accompany your significant other to a local steak

house for dinner. You order a 9 ounce sirloin, and for your two

side orders you select two orders of broccoli, and request regular

butter for the broccoli. You have unsweetened iced tea to drink.

Skip the hot bread they put on the table ... if your partner doesn't

mind, ask them not to bring it at all. Besides the bill, the price of

your trip to the steak joint is:

FOOD	SERVING SIZE	TOTAL CARBS	TOTAL FIBER	NET CARBS
Sirloin Steak	9 oz.	0	0	0
Broccoli	1 cup	6	2	4
Iced Tea	2 glasses	0	0	0
Artificial Sweetener	1 packet	0	0	0
TOTALS		6	2	4

Table 4.3

Tonight you really want a little dessert, so when you get home, you have something small ... say an Atkins desert bar. You eat a pack of the Atkins Peanut Butter Cups ... if you close your eyes you can almost imagine it being some Reese's Cups! Add the following to your carb totals:

FOOD	SERV SIZE	CARBS	FIBER	SUGAR ALCOHOLS	NET CARBS
Atkins Peanut Butter Cups	2 pieces	18	5	11	2
TOTALS		18	5	11	2

Table 4.4

You don't have to be a math major to see that you have eaten about 16 *net carbohydrates* worth of food today, which is well below your 30 net carbohydrate limit. You may have wanted to have some almonds or cheese as a snack during the day ... if so, calculate the net carbohydrates and add them into your total. Most days you will find it's kind of hard to reach 30 net carbohydrates. So, in a nutshell, that is how this stuff works ... simple, but not always easy to do.

Don't get nervous ... certainly the meals I have listed here are not the only things you can eat. Know that nearly all foods have carbohydrates, and it is your duty to check the carbohydrate numbers of everything you eat BEFORE you pop it in your mouth. And I mean EVERYTHING! There are so many foods with hidden carbohydrates that you must ... must ... must check the nutrition information on everything. A great example is that I was taking a chewable Vitamin C supplement for a few years before I thought to check its components. I was stunned to note that it had 5 carbohydrates per pill. So I now take a different type that is 2 carbohydrates. Over the course of the day, if you can chop out a number of carbohydrates just by paying attention, it will be to your benefit.

As for checking the nutrition information for your food, most of us know that the government has requirements for listing the numbers on the various packages. In addition, there are many free apps for your computer or smart phone that can give you all the nutrition info that you seek ... if you have them on your phone they are accessible at all times. A word of advice ... in addition to an app as a general resource, find one that lists nutritional info for all the restaurant chains as well. If you get caught at a restaurant, a quick glance at a restaurant app will give you the facts you need to make an educated food choice.

Finally, I mentioned earlier that folks complain because they have to *count* carbohydrates. I can't believe that in the scope of a person's life, spending just a moment to check some carbohydrate and fiber numbers is a big deal. As bodybuilder Dave Draper (2001) noted, *"Can we intelligently argue that our daily obligations are more important than our health? It is our health, ultimately, about which we speak: body, mind and soul."* I agree, so lose this lame excuse. The carbohydrate count in whatever you ingest is your measuring stick … it's the way you'll stay on track. It takes only a few seconds to do, and after a very short time, you won't need to do it often, since you will know what you can eat and what you can't. If you want to occasionally verify how you are doing, count your carbohydrates daily for a week … if you are making any errors, this will bring them to your attention. But please don't try to justify not following this plan because you have to look on the back of a few packages for a couple of numbers … you would essentially be sabotaging your health and your future.

The Diet and Fiber Intake

It is no secret that for your body's wellness, fiber is mandatory. Regarding our ancestors again, when guys and gals were first walking around upright, munching on meat, they ate the nuts, leaves, and berries that were high in fiber. As we evolved, our diets have changed too, and not necessarily for the better. Today's average person only gets about half of their daily fiber needs. To make matters worse, that 50% number reflects those that aren't on a restrictive diet of some sort ... the numbers for those folks are even worse. It is crucial to examine fiber and its relative importance to your body.

We begin your quick class on fiber with the fact that fiber is generally divided into two types: *soluble* (dissolves in water) and *insoluble* (does not easily dissolve in water). Soluble fiber can be found in a number of sources, including beans, oats / oat cereals, seeds, dark leafy vegetables, and nuts. Soluble fibers will absorb water as they enter your digestive system, resulting in formation of a paste, which in turn slows digestion. This serves to help you feel full. It will also attach to particles of cholesterol and remove them from the body. Insoluble fiber does not absorb water, and in fact passes through the body basically unchanged. It adds bulk to your diet, and by doing so helps the body fight constipation by making the stool softer and heavier. Found mainly in fruits (particularly in the seeds and skins) and in whole grains, insoluble fiber acts as a natural laxative that helps to keep the inside of your pipes cleaned out.

From a reduced carbohydrate perspective, most fiber is actually *high* in carbohydrates, but since it is passed through the body without changing state, the glucose release is not accomplished. This eliminates the need for the body's insulin to fluctuate in an effort to counteract it. This is the primary reason that we can safely subtract the "fiber count" out of our total carbohydrates when following a net carbohydrate plan.

How does fiber affect the obese? As I have noted elsewhere in this book, diets most often fail due to the participant being hungry. Fiber helps to combat hunger, since by its nature it adds bulk and is more dense, contributing to the feeling of being full ... or at least not empty! In short, in addition to all the internal positives acquired from fiber, it also helps to blunt the hunger response in the body.

So, in summation ... FIBER IS GOOD! Adult women should ingest between 25 - 30 grams of fiber per day, while adult men should shoot for between 30 - 35 grams. Fiber serves to reduce hunger ... increases transport of waste through the body ... reduces constipation ... helps the body avoid diverticulitis, colitis, and cancer ... combats hemorrhoids ... and has any number of other positive results. One thing to note is that the addition of fiber alone will not cause you to lose weight, and should be paired with a change in eating to accomplish weight loss. It also pays to use caution with both your choice and amount of fiber, since you could end up being much, much gassier ... no way to make friends!

What About Other Diets?

There are as many different types of eating plans out there as there are snowflakes, but they are generally based on either limiting calories or limiting fat. These diets generally fail due to one common problem ... hunger.

Nobody knows the tremendous long term failure rate of these diets more than obese folks. The self discipline needed to lose weight by reducing calories or fat is astronomical. There is usually some amount of success for a short time, but often fails over the long haul. The reason is quite simple ... people stay hungry all the time on most diets. I myself struggled through all of these problems in my journey. I must have started trying to lose weight by reducing calories and / or fat at least 20 times in my life. During those attempts, I would find myself hungry shortly after I ate, and for awhile I would beat the feeling. Inevitably, whether it was days, weeks, or months, I would always fail. And it was simply because I was always hungry. To make matters worse, I didn't understand at that time that I was torpedoing myself constantly by eating "good food" like potatoes, pasta, etc. which screwed with my insulin level, leaving me constantly craving more food. I'll never forget sitting down with a plate of celery sticks and thinking ... really? For the rest of my life? I think not. An eating plan is only successful if you can follow it.

Climbing on my soapbox for a moment ... quite frankly, I'm a little angry at the government for their backing of these types of diets. Where does it say that our diets should follow a "food pyramid" loaded with carbohydrates? I firmly think that the government (and many others) said that crap so much that they started believing it. After awhile, the average fatty out there like me figured that their research MUST have proven this to be true, so it must be the right path to take. Again, I can safely call BULL.

It is also pretty obvious that a lot of companies have made (and continue to make) loads of money providing diet alternatives for the masses. There are countless different options on the market ... you see them advertised on television all hours of the day and night. They each have a different approach, but as an interesting side note, I have noticed that over the past few years that most of these plans have begun to offer programs based on the "glycemic index", which is of course a fancy way to say reducing carbohydrates. Each plan has its own pros and cons, but in summation, the general downfalls are price and inconvenience. Regardless of what plan you're tempted to follow, just remember that on the far end you still need to have learned to eat properly for the rest of your life ... so while many people do okay while they are "on" one of these plans, they will crash and burn after they "leave the nest" to fend for themselves. I prefer to give folks a method that works the same at the beginning as it does years later. I find that KISS (*Keep It Simple Stupid*) works well, and by choosing to follow the ideas in this book, you can take control of your own future. No weigh-ins, no food deliveries from the UPS guy, no pills, no shots. You are in charge of your success without the structure and cost of an outside support mechanism. However, the plan in this book also removes the crutch, and requires you to be responsible and accountable ... to yourself.

Beware the Low Carb Flu

As you have no doubt deciphered along the way, I am a true believer in low carbohydrate eating ... many of the reasons are listed in this book. However, because I owe you complete disclosure, I feel that I must mention to you one particularly malicious byproduct of this low carbohydrate living. The sneaky offender? The *low carb flu!*

If you recall, we discussed that by limiting your carbohydrate intake, the body would be forced to search elsewhere for a fuel to burn. By now, you also understand that if glucose isn't available, our internal engines will start to burn fats instead. As the body starts to burn fats, it begins to shift towards something that the really smart scientific types call *ketosis*. Ummm, ketosis is some sort of metabolic magic that occurs when the liver does something to some sort of molecules ... but that is WAY past the level of the author of this book! Feel free to dig up more information on the subject if you dare. For our benefit here, just know that ketosis is the goal for low carbohydrate eaters, since it indicates that you have successfully made the big switch in fuel from carbohydrates (actually glucose) to fats. Oh, and as a byproduct of torching the fats and reaching ketosis, the body produces ... you guessed it ... *ketones*.

Finally, after all the years of feeding your body sugars for fuel, you asked it (actually, forced it) to start burning fats instead. Great start on your part. However, for many people this change in fuel sources ... and the subsequent arrival in ketosis ... is often accompanied by a general lethargic state fondly referred to as the *low carb flu*. I didn't name it, but it is definitely real! The symptoms vary for different folks, but generally include headaches, irritability, exhaustion, and just feeling generally crappy. Having been a shift worker for years, the foggy and hazy feeling you get from this "flu" is very similar to the feeling you have the day after you work your first midnight shift! Oh, even though I mentioned you would likely get a headache, I'm mentioning it again here just because I feel I need to ... headache probability is high!

This discomfort is nothing more than a gift of metabolic punishment from your body, which is trying to bully you back into eating carbohydrates. But stand strong ... don't give in! Know that some people barely notice it, while others take a couple of weeks to get past it. Probably 90 percent of people that I know that started a low carbohydrate eating plan feel the effects for around three days, then it passes. When it does, most folks have a new energy level that was higher than before they began to change their food intake.

There are a few things that may help you mitigate the severity of the symptoms. Drink extra water, since it will hydrate you as well as flush out the byproducts of the fuel swap (namely ketones). In fact, if you have planned the start date of your new eating plan, it wouldn't hurt to increase your water intake several days ahead. Also, if you take supplements, don't forget them. Although I don't often recommend skipping your workouts, during this time it wouldn't be a bad thing to scale them back for a few days until your energy level returns. Finally, become friends with your over the counter pain killer of choice ... whether you prefer ibuprofen, acetaminophen, aspirin, or some other *legal* pain reducer, keep some of it handy. The important thing to take away from this feeling is that it is natural, normal, and a signal that your body is changing ... it will pass.

Personally...

You know you have achieved the place you want to be when you can look at food as just fuel for your engine, which of course in this case is your body. However, many people still have some kind of emotional attachment to food. Below are several of the most common excuses I hear when discussing reduced carbohydrate eating with people ... and my typical response as well!

Comment: "You know, this diet isn't for everyone"
Bruce: "You're right, it's only a diet for folks who want to lose weight and keep it off for life"

Comment: "The best way to lose weight is to eat the same foods you always eat, but just eat less of it"
Bruce: Sure ... and that is like telling an alcoholic *I know you're an alcoholic, so we're going to cure you by having you drink the same booze you always drink, but just drink less of it.* Uh, yep ... that sounds like a recipe for success.

Comment: "You have to live a little bit too."
Bruce: This eating style will allow you to do just that ... *live.*

5   WORKOUT

*"Those who think they have not time for bodily exercise
will sooner or later have to find time for illness."*
Edward Stanley (British Statesman)

Workout (General Info)

I know ... you're ready to read all about how to work out to
help you achieve wellness. Slow down ... I promise its coming. I
have some other brilliant stuff to tell you first. Just a reminder ...
by now I hope you have made the decision to check in with your
regular doctor to get their okay to start a new eating and workout
plan. If you don't have a regular doctor, I say again ... GET ONE!
It is critical that you develop a relationship with a physician, not
to mention just plain common sense. Nowww we can go on to the
workout stuff!

I think most of you will agree that the body is an amazing
machine. At its core, the express purpose of our "machine" is to
perform work to keep us alive. Our distant ancestor's day
consisted of running around killing dinosaurs, and trying to keep
their bodies from becoming groceries for any number of
predators. Basically, they consumed their entire days with just
trying to stay alive. They relied heavily on their physical prowess
to achieve this, and the ones who couldn't keep up became
examples for the *survival of the fittest* adage! As the generations
continued to die off and others were born, mankind gradually
found ways to make daily life easier.

Throughout history, many inventions were the result of the search for labor saving devices. Let's face it ... putting clothes in a washing machine in your laundry room is much easier than hauling them to the river and beating them with rocks. The next time you turn on the stove, imagine having to gather or chop wood to cook with. My wife's Italian grandfather would tell stories of the women in Italy walking into the mountains to pick up firewood ... when they had all they could possibly carry on their backs, they would bring it back into town and sell it ... as he would say, "for one cents per bundle"! In my younger years, I myself spent many long, hot Florida days in fields hoisting hundreds of hay bales onto trucks, then taking them back to barns and unloading them. These bales weighed around 60 pounds ... unless it rained, when they would weigh well over 100 pounds. Um, okay Bruce, come back off of the farm ... where are you going with this? I guess you could say that the labor saving devices have worked, because the majority of people don't do as much physical labor as they used to. While that can be considered progress, we must remember that our body is designed to do work. So, to keep the body at any appreciable level of physical proficiency, we must perform some amount of work. If you don't get much physical labor as part of your normal daily duties, then you have got to find other ways to challenge the body.

Because the reader of this book is likely overweight (at the very least), then the challenge for them becomes to find or design a work out that will increase their basic strength and aerobic capacity while burning calories ... in short, working within their limitations to increase their physical wellness. As I stated earlier, it is my experience that reaching an increased fitness level results from about sixty percent dietary changes, with the other forty percent from workouts. By now I hope you have absorbed the dietary and weight loss information from the previous chapter, and have made a commitment to change your eating patterns. Likewise, in the upcoming Wellness chapter you will be presented with evidence that working out / physical wellness is a huge contributing factor to the health of your entire being. However, for now, our concentration should be on following a regular workout program, since this is a conduit through which you can accelerate weight loss, as well as firm, tone, and shape your body. I am here to help ... read on!

Excuses, Excuses

I really don't think there is a person in any developed country who doesn't realize the importance of working out for health. It is no surprise that a structured workout will burn calories, strengthen muscles, increase bone density, increase metabolic rate, and about a million other things.

Armed with that knowledge, you would think that people would race to the gym to get started. However, as our history has proven, mankind is very adaptable, and in this case they have adapted by perfecting the art of *excuse making* to justify why they *don't* work out. I would like to address the most common of these reasons to bail out on exercise, and by doing so hopefully spur you to begin a regular workout program.

The most prevalent alibi for bailing out on a work out is "I'm just too busy." Maybe you should sit down before I address this one ... prepare yourself for possibly the biggest understatement you will read in this book. Are you ready ... here it is ... *people lead busy lives*. That was it? C'mon Bruce, everybody knows that. That's really weak ... give us something more than that. Okay, I will.

I agree that people are busy today. In fact, I propose that they are busier than at any time in history. While their lives are easier physically than those of their ancestors, those same lives are simultaneously much more complex. The amount of decisions to be made during the day, as well as the amount of information that needs to be processed, have increased exponentially through the years. There can be no doubt that this impinges on personal free time in ways never before encountered. Sometimes this time crunch is due to circumstances beyond their control, while in other instances it may be a result of their own choices. Regardless, for the purposes of this book, I want to stipulate that people are very busy ... and they are equally eager to use their schedule as a crutch for not exercising regularly. If you have ever said (or heard someone say) "I would love to work out, but I'm just too busy to get to the gym", I say ... Arnold Schwarzennegger. Huh? What does a bodybuilder ... turned movie star ... turned governor of California ... turned back into actor ... have to do with this? I'm glad you asked.

In the early 1980s, a new fitness facility was opening in the city where I lived, and Arnold was the guest speaker. Of course, this was just after the release of his newest movie Conan the Barbarian ... and long before his political aspirations would come true. No, at this time he was just AHHNOLD ... bodybuilder extraordinaire. Sure enough, my wife and I attended the seminar, and one question he was asked was "with jobs, etc., can the average guy become a competitive bodybuilder?" He chuckled, and said a few things about genetics, then he got to the point he wanted to make. He said that everyone should remember that there are "TVENTY-FOUR OWAS IN EVRY DAY", and not to get caught up in the "normal." He related the story that when he and bodybuilding partner Franco Columbo had first come to this country, they had small stipends from some bodybuilding moguls, but that they still needed to work to make ends meet. So they would go to the gym for 1 1/2 hours early in the morning, then head to work all day laying bricks and other associated mason work. After work, they would generally come home, take a nap, then return to the gym for another workout. Of course, Arnold being Arnold, he said they would then go out and PAHHTY and chase GURRLS. Along the way, Arnold and Franco would open other businesses as well as getting college educations; Arnold received a business degree and Franco became a chiropractor. Yet on the day that I saw him in person, his central point was that there are 24 hours in each day, so don't get caught up with thinking that you HAVE TO work the same hours every day, sleep the same hours each night, and so on. Make good use of your time.

   With that story in mind, I say to you yet again that everyone has a busy schedule. In fact, most of us think we just can't fit another thing in. I propose to you that you may need to change your thought process. You *need to create the time to exercise*. Quite frankly, I can promise you that the person with your best interest at heart is ... you! No one on this planet cares more for you than you do. You MUST make time for you. As it relates to your workouts, they must become part of your routine, like brushing your teeth.

When to Work Out

With my brilliant recounting of Arnold still fresh in your mind, I know you are asking yourself ... *after fifty years why can't Arnold lose the accent and speak better English?"* Ooops ... I meant, you were wondering "when is the best time of day for me to work out?" Since you have turned to my book for help, I'll definitively answer your question by saying ... I don't have a clue! There are so many personal variables involved in making that decision that it is impossible for me to counsel you!

Generally speaking, the majority of people work out in the afternoon or early evening following their daily commitment to work, school, family duties, etc. While this is primarily due to convenience, there is some science to support that later workouts are better. The body core temperature is at its highest, hormones and testosterone are usually higher, and quite frankly, most folks are stronger in the afternoon.

As for me, I am a "morning person" and typically hit the gym around 06:30 in the morning. I happen to like starting my day with a workout, since it sort of revs me up, as well as gives me the knowledge that no matter what occurs the rest of the day, I was able to get my workout in. I am certain that I am slightly weaker in the morning, but I am willing to concede that. As a veteran of rotating shift work, I have literally trained at all hours of the day, and I can tell you that no particular time was the perfect answer. As Draper (2001) notes, *"Each workout is a unique and separate experience unto itself. Events of the day, mood, energy levels and tensions affect every performance differently."* Bravo, Dave. Every workout will not contain personal records. The important thing is that for weight loss and control ... as well as for your overall physical wellness ... you need to perform some sort of activity regardless of the reading on the clock. Whether you are able to maintain a regular workout schedule, or if your schedule necessitates that you alternate your workout to various days or times, the important point to be made is that you MUST find time to push your body. After all, aren't you worth it?

Where to Work Out

With the issue of *when* to work out behind us, it is important to know that many, many people still struggle with the question of *where* to work out. When asked, I often answer that a workout can be found anywhere, and in any number of ways. However, for the benefit of this book, we will assume that we are trying to decide between the traditional choice of working out at home or in a gym. Possibly the best thing to do is analyze your situation to see what is the best fit. What are your goals, your limitations, that sort of thing. It's also nice for you to know that you aren't the only one wrestling with this decision. I'll try my best to address the pros and cons of both. At the risk of being labeled Captain Obvious, while passing along this info, hopefully I will give you a little more food for thought to help you make your decision.

Working Out at Home

Many people choose to work out at home, and there are a number of valid reasons that support that choice. These choices seem to break down into one of three categories: financial, psychological, or convenience.

The primary reason that most folks choose to work out at home is the cost savings ... working out at home avoids the gym membership fees. Memberships are a fact of life in a gym, since the gym owner has to cover their costs and make a few bucks too. There are as many gym pricing packages as there are stars in the sky, and generally you can find one that fits your needs. However, if you know without a doubt that your budget cannot handle another cost, then this eliminates gyms.

Ranking a close second place behind costs are the psychological qualms about going to a gym. You might feel that you look stupid trying to figure out all the machines and contraptions in a gym. Possibly you think that you "jiggle" too much when using the cardio equipment. Of course, there's always the anxiety you feel when you walk into the gym wearing your brand new [INSERT NAME BRAND HERE] workout gear. You could just be an introverted personality whose circuits overload in a crowd. Regardless of the cause your angst, you quiver at the thought of working out in public. (I'll have more on this later). Hello, home workouts.

Finally, there is the convenience factor. It seems that there are a variety of gyms opening in nearly every city. Some are big, corporate facilities with pools, saunas, equipment, and classes. Others may be the quick, in and out facilities. Still others may be the mom and pop style. Obviously, with this competition, the consumer has more choices in business hours, locations, and amenities. Yet, if the gyms that are in your area don't offer what you need, it doesn't make sense for you to join ... your home gym will be available around the clock.

There are other contributing considerations for working out at home. Certainly, along with twenty four hour a day access and no extra driving needed, it is a fact that during your home workouts the equipment is never busy. You can set up training circuits without someone else jumping in. Whether your workout music leans toward Metallica or Mozart, you can always enjoy your choice of tunes (volume options depend on your audio equipment and the tolerance of your neighbors). Not to be downplayed, if you rank somewhere between "just a little squeamish about hygiene" and a full blown *mysophobic* (fearful of germs), at home the only perspiration on your equipment will be yours!

As with everything in life, there is always the other side. There are some notable negatives in your quest for fitness at home. The cost of all the equipment needed can be significant, depending on your needs. And if you want a good variety of equipment, space can quickly become a stumbling block. Most notably, life often gets in the way. There always seems to be something tugging at you when you're at home, whether it's the telephone ringing, kids hollering, visitors stopping by, the cat throwing up a hairball, or a hundred other things. Whether it is caused by intrinsic or extrinsic factors, lack of motivation can become a real problem with home workouts.

Working Out at a Gym

In the United States in 2015, more than 64 million people were health club members, representing a growth of 22% since 2009 (IHRSA, 2016). That means roughly one person out of five in the U.S. belongs to a gym. It seems gym membership is an example of people speaking with their wallets! The question arises, why do people prefer going to a gym?

By joining a gym, you immediately have access to a wide variety of equipment and services. It is not unusual for a good sized workout facility to be 20,000 square feet or bigger, using that space for equipment, classrooms, courts, pools, locker rooms, showers, or any number of other amenities. Most gyms offer child care at least during the busiest hours. In addition, you will inevitably have the ability to interact with trainers about any of your questions. Last, and certainly not least, there is normally a staff of janitorial and cleaning personnel working to keep the place clean!

Beside the physical facilities, the gym offers you a number of other benefits. For instance, gyms offer an outlet for social interaction. Gyms are full of people who have a common goal; the goal is fitness. Yet regardless of their goals and the level of fitness they desire, they are all people. The gym visit can function as a social boost for you as well. Please don't think I mean you should sit on the machines and talk while others are waiting! My point is that by interacting with others, you may find someone to work out with. You may ask someone to spot you on an exercise for safety. There is no doubt you will see someone doing an exercise that you don't recognize, so ask them about it ... but wait until they finish! You may prefer to just put the ear buds in your ears and enjoy the solace of music and a workout. Plus, while not everyone is lookin' for love at the gym, it is undoubtedly a social atmosphere ... one survey finds that three out of four people prefer to meet someone at the gym than at a bar. So, if you need to strengthen your social wellness, don't forget about the possibilities at a gym.

Finally, the last thing to point out is that the gym offers a combination of less distractions and more motivation. All of the famous distractions we mentioned in our home workout section above are not a problem at the gym. Regardless of how busy the rest of your life is, in your gym you can close out the outside world and concentrate on your workout. Which leads back to the motivation part. Gyms have every type of person as members, with a wide variety of sizes, shapes, ages, and any other demographic you can imagine. The result is an automatic buzz that happens inside a gym. People are pushing, pulling, straining, running, and anything else that leads to increasing their physical wellness. The buzz that permeates a gym is often palpable, and its impact is beneficial.

There are many times that you may have had a tough day ... you're tired and actually want to just go home. You force your car into the gym parking lot ... you know that you really should go in ... okay, you'll go in, but you are certain that you aren't going to do much when you get inside. You drag in, change clothes in the locker room, then slink into the gym looking like an inmate headed for the electric chair. As you begin to warm up, despite your mood you can feel some of the day's stress begin to leave. As you continue to work out, the atmosphere around you picks you up like a surfer on a wave. You suddenly find yourself going a little heavier on the weights, or a little faster on that exercise bike, or pushing the "incline" arrow up on the treadmill more than usual. Just the act of getting into the gym served to pick you up.

Motivation can come in many ways. As a long time gym patron, I have seen all types of people working out: folks with missing or prosthetic limbs, people confined to wheelchairs, the arthritic, the very old. None of them are asking for anything, they are just there to work out. If I'm having a bad day and see one of them working out despite the stumbling blocks in front of them, it motivates me ... and tells me to quit whining. Just today, I spoke to a man at the gym who happened to be 92 years old. He is slightly unsteady on his feet, but he comes to the gym six days a week. I asked how he was, and he said he felt like he was slowing down! By the way, he still drives, and actually delivers Meals on Wheels during the week.

Heck, one time, without realizing it, I was even the one

giving inspiration! I had a stress fracture in one of my feet, forcing me to wear a soft cast up to my knee for 12 weeks. Although I still wanted to get my workouts in, I didn't want to hobble around and get in other folks way. So instead of my normal early morning program when the gym was fairly busy, I would go to the gym around 1:00 in the afternoon, traditionally one of the least busy times in any gym. As the weeks passed, I would see the same small crowd on a regular basis. Eventually, my foot healed and I finally was able to remove the cast. I was in the gym one afternoon (sans cast) and a young man in his mid 30s stopped and spoke. He noticed my cast was off, and just wanted to tell me that when he would feel like cutting his workout short, he would look at me working with my leg in a cast and it would motivate him to continue. He said it was "cool" to see someone with a cast on but working out so hard. I told him I appreciated it ... and also said that I hoped to never provide any more motivation with any other broken body parts! So you never know where you will find your motivation ... or if you might accidentally become someone else's.

As a means of wrapping all this together, earlier we mentioned that one reason so many choose to work out at home instead of a gym is that they are self conscious ... in fact, many say that they are too embarrassed to go to a gym due to their physical condition. This one drives me crazy. One of the underlying themes of this book is that you need to take charge of your life ...

FOR YOU. In keeping with that theory, do not let the fact that you aren't currently a magazine model stop you from going to a gym. For goodness sake, you have made the decision to increase your wellness, so grab it and shake it! Who cares what others think about you? You aren't working out for them ... you are doing it for your own well being. Frankly, you may be surprised at the outpouring of support you may receive from others in the gym. I know that if I see someone who is challenged in any way (age, weight, physical handicap, etc.) I generally make an effort to congratulate them on their efforts. Please understand that most people will see you the first time you come in, but after that they don't really give you a second thought. It kind of reminds me of Cesar Milan (*The Dog Whisperer*) when he brings a new dog into his pack ... after the dogs all introduce themselves by sniffing each other's butt, they go on about their business. I'm praying that this analogy doesn't give you too many upsetting mental images ... and I am certainly not suggesting you employ non-traditional greeting methods in the gym. The point to be made is *get over yourself and work out.*

What to Wear

Since I am in my sixth decade on earth, I have been around the workout and gym scene for many years. I was around when people thought that strength training was weird, and it was a "well known fact" that weight training only slowed you down. I remember that the Sears 110 pound, cement filled plastic weight sets were found in most every garage. At that time you were more apt to see homemade benches than anything from a manufacturer. Of course, through the early 1970s, commercial gyms were nothing like what you see today. Not a single gym I ever saw then had more than 60 percent of its lights working, leaving them dark and ominous. These dingy palaces also possessed a certain unique kind of aroma that was easily perceptible through the front door ... which was always hanging open. It was sort of a sweaty high school locker room bouquet, occasionally tempered with a splash of bleach or pine cleaner. They were full of shaky, rusty, often homemade equipment. Padded surfaces of any bench wore always wore copious amounts of tape to cover the splits ... variety of tape not important. Invariably, in at least one corner of the gym were old kettle bells or Indian clubs (those bowling pin things), standing as stark reminders of the strength training of old. Oh, and don't forget the proprietor. He was always an older guy in a "wife beater" t-shirt, sporting gnarled fingers, big knuckles, and a gravelly voice. Invariably he was an old boxer ... or wrestler ... or trainer. Oh, he

72

was also not shy at all about sticking his finger in your chest and discussing with you the fact that you left some of your weights on the bar or broke some other gym etiquette.

Contrast this with today's clean, well lit facilities, all full of shiny whatzits, barbells, dumbbells and benches of all types, and with aerobic equipment stretching from the front door to the horizon! Not to mention, there is a Misty or Heather at the front desk, ready to give you a tour and talk to you about the schedule for spinning and yoga!

However, despite these monumental changes, there is one transformation that is more mind boggling to me than all the rest. That is … I cannot believe the amount of thought (and money) people will invest in their gym attire! I never gave this any thought until somewhere around the early 1980s, when physical fitness met marketing. Olivia Newton John made her famous "Physical" video, and the rest was history! It wasn't enough that women were now starting to train in the same gyms as men, but fashion became as important as the workout itself!

Now, I operate under the theory that your workout clothes should fit and be comfortable. If you are okay in a pair of cotton shorts and t-shirt (as I am) it's okay to wear that. Your performance won't suffer, and you will be just fine. I do advise you not to wear clothing three sizes too big, since it will become a hindrance when you sweat. It will hang off of you and invariably get wound up or hung on something as you try to work out. So, get some stuff that fits. Suitable shoes are very important, so don't skimp in that department. Go somewhere and get your feet measured so that you know what size shoe you should buy. Yes ladies, this means you ... I hazard a guess that half the women I have known wear the wrong size shoes! Don't fret that someone will call you Sasquatch if you get the right size. As your fitness level increases, you may even begin to run. At that time, you may want to consider buying running shoes as well, since they are more flexible and designed to withstand more impact. However, for our scenario here, I envision that a good walking or cross training shoe will suit your requirements for quite a while. Remember, when it comes to workout gear, fit is better than fancy. Athletic clothing comes in any size, and basic is fine.

The power of marketing is best illustrated by an experience that I had recently in my gym. Before I begin my workouts, I loosen up my body by spending about 10 minutes on either the treadmill, exercise bike, or elliptical machine, and then go through some light lifting and pressing on a cable machine to stretch my body. While I was on the treadmill, I happened to notice a guy enter the gym. He had matching workout shorts and shirt (from a major name brand apparel company), and I watched intently as he donned his weightlifting gloves, strapped on his combination music device / heart rate / pulse monitor onto his upper arm. He produced a weight belt out of nowhere, and cinched it up. I thought that this guy was going to war. Then, he blew the air loudly out of his lungs a couple of times, and eased into a lat pull down machine. He set the weight, reared back, and performed 8 blistering repetitions with 30 pounds on the machine! Now, I give him thumbs up for being in the gym, and I certainly don't know if he had any underlying physical / medical issues that precluded him from doing anything further. However, it is most likely that he succumbed to the advertising / marketing industry, and purchased every piece of gear he could find. If you want to deck yourself out in such an outfit, feel free, but note that it doesn't mean you will suddenly start working out harder. Just be sure to wear something that fits.

Aches and Pains

With my body, I would NEVER, EVER, EVER be confused with a prima ballerina. I am much more likely to be compared to a Clydesdale than a graceful dancer. So it is with all the admiration I can muster that I relate to you a wonderful quote from famed ballet prodigy Mikhail Baryshnikov, who aptly noted that *the more injuries you get, the smarter you get.* Whether you're a ballet fan or not, please know that this is an amazingly accurate statement!

As you embark on your physical wellness journey, it is important to know that over time, you will most definitely encounter the aches and pains of your body changing its ways. I often tell people that at my age I am going to be sore anyway, so at least if I'm working out I know what caused it! One of the most basic things to understand is that you need to be in touch with your body so that you are able to answer the inevitable question ... "Are you hurt or are you injured?"

Those of you who have a penchant for watching less than fantastic movies may recognize this quote from the less than fantastic football movie "The Program." In the movie, a football player was down on the field with some sort of leg injury, and was asked by his coach (actor James Caan) if he was *hurt* or *injured.* Caan would clarify by saying that "if you're injured, I can't let you go back in, but if you are hurt then you can play." By the way, this response typified the deep, philosophical underpinnings of this movie ... ummm, not really, it just showed a coach trying to get a running back to go back in the game! But it is a valid synopsis for comparison sake. I think of the difference between *hurt* and *injured* as the aftermath of smacking your hand with a hammer. If you dance around for a few moments, saying words you probably shouldn't be saying, you are most likely hurt. If you can't even curse, need to go to get x-rays, and end up with a cast, you are injured.

It is almost a certainty that you will encounter aches and pains resulting from your workouts. It is important to learn and understand your body so that you can differentiate between the states of "hurt" and "injured." If you can't tell, go visit your physician. One other point ... a question lots of folks have is about whether to work out when they are sick. We all get colds, coughs, and the flu, and every time it is different. While it's impossible to make a blanket statement about working out while sick, there is a rule of thumb that says if you're sick from the neck up, you can probably work out. If you're sick from the neck down, it's probably best to skip the workouts until you feel better. I guess that means a head cold is not really going to get worse if you work out, while working out with bronchitis in the lungs may cause you more harm than good. Be smart ... listen to your body.

Remember the RICE

If I would have gone to my medical professional for every discomfort during the last 45 years or so, it would have cost me enough that I could pay off the United States' deficit! For many exercise induced pains, it is important to know that you can usually apply a self-administered first aid method known by the mnemonic RICE, which stands for *Rest, Ice, Compression, and Elevation.*

- Rest ... if you find yourself pretty sore, it is in your best interest to rest so that your body can begin to repair itself. If you continue to stress the injured area it will only lead to more inflammation and pain, and even worse damage. Generally speaking, rest enough so that the affected area has the majority of function returned and most of the pain is gone.

- Ice ... it functions as nature's anti-inflammatory. Injured areas have increased heat levels due to increased blood flow, causing inflammation. Applying ice removes this heat, stops inflammation, and reduces swelling. I use ice by placing a moist washcloth on top of the injury, then placing an ice pack (or sandwich bag) full of ice on top of the washcloth. Of course, the washcloth prevents frostbite or other skin issues. Best recommendation here is to apply

78

the ice for 20 minutes, removing for 20 minutes, then repeat as often as possible up to 48 hours after the injury.

- Compression ... will help to control / reduce the swelling from the inflammation resulting from injury. Swelling is the enemy, causing pain, stiffness, and loss of function. Placing an elastic type bandage on the area ... snug enough not to allow free movement, but not so tight to limit circulation ... will help to compress and support the area, which in turn will manage the swelling and enable the area to heal quicker.

- Elevation ... helps to reduce swelling by using gravity. If the injured area is elevated (particularly above the level of the heart) gravity helps to transport fluid away from the injury, reducing swelling.

As always, if in doubt about the extent of your injuries, have the doc check you out. However, by using the simple steps of RICE you may alleviate many common maladies that you encounter as you push your body.

Oh ... and after you use RICE for up to 48 hours to stop any further inflammation of your injury, you may also consider using heat therapy. The opposite of cold temperatures that are used to slow down the blood flow, heat therapy will open up the vessels, increasing blood supply ... and bringing with it nutrients and oxygen to help with muscle aches and stiffness. While the heat can be either dry or moist, in my experience moist heat is superior in loosening up the body. Moist heat is applied using several methods, including warm showers and baths, hot water bottles, and gel packs. However, the most effective way I found to apply moist heat is to use an electric heating pad, with a damp cloth or towel between the heating pad and your skin. The advantage of the electric pad is that you can set the temperature and it will stay fairly constant. To use it properly, set the pad to a warm setting, apply to the damp cloth over the injured area, then apply the warm heating pad to the cloth following the 20 minutes on, 20 minutes off schedule similar to ice therapy. Heat therapy is not only for injury rehabilitation, but can also effective for the average sore, stiff muscles.

How to Work Out

Enough of the preliminaries ... now it's time to address the 800 pound gorilla in the room. So far in our book, it has been proposed, insinuated, implied, hinted, and suggested that physical activity has magical properties when it comes to health and wellness. Well, it does. The supporting evidence is overwhelming ... *physical activity is vital and correlates directly to better health.* Based on your inner willpower (as well as this persuasive book!), you are finally ready to commit to some sort of workout plan to contribute to your wellness. Immediately, the question becomes *how exactly can this be accomplished*? Especially if you are overweight, obese, or even morbidly obese?

First, know that *knowledge is power.* I'm robbing this quote from Sir Francis Bacon, English philosopher, statesman, scientist, jurist, orator, and author. My literary theft is based on the premise that because of my many years of having worked out ... as well as lots and lots of studying about working out ... and having made a few workout mistakes in that time ... there are some things I can pass along to you for your consideration.

First, as a friendly suggestion, I wholeheartedly propose that you get your eating program started and under control before you begin a structured workout regimen. Don't get excited ... I mean just delay the regimented, controlled workouts for maybe a couple of weeks. Honestly, it is my experience that most folks only have enough stamina and mental discipline to gather all their resources to fight one thing at a time. Change your eating habits first, and you will have more energy physically ... as well as be "pumped" as you notice weight loss. Remember, there is such a thing as the "bad snowball" effect of being overweight and tired ... which makes you not want to exert any energy ... which in turn makes you more tired and overweight. I submit that this is probably where many of those reading this book are at right now. The great news is that the inverse is also true, since as you lose weight, your energy levels increase and you prefer to be more active as a result.

Before we go any further down this road, I want to stress that being active throughout your day is vitally important to achieving weight loss and increases in wellness. Washing the car, mowing the grass, parking a little further away from the store ... this hidden exercise is a great way to increase your fitness level. However, for our benefit, I want to consider workouts as being those scheduled blocks of time that you can devote strictly to working out. Regardless of your choice of location, during a structured session you can much more successfully track and monitor the response of your body to the exercise. I feel this ability to observe the reaction of your body is vital ... particularly early in the process of changing your body composition and habits. As an example, if you walk for 20 minutes on a treadmill, you can closely observe your heart rate, and manipulate it by changing treadmill intensity (speed, incline, etc.). As I said, washing the car is great too, but as an activity, it is tough to quantify / qualify your results ... well, except that your car looks better! So, for the rest of this Workout section, let's assume that the action takes place within a structured workout regimen.

Moving forward, we will examine exercise in a little better detail, keeping the big folks in mind. While designing any exercise program can be as involved or as simple as you would like to make it, two things are blatantly obvious. First, it is the logical and sensible thing to plan a program that is both safe and effective. Second, the most important thing to remember is to *move* ... being overweight is bad, but being overweight and sedentary is much, much worse.

Equally important is to understand that many of those non-obese folks among us can't really appreciate the self-limiting properties of obesity. It is easy for others to take for granted things like being able to reach down and tie their shoes ... or getting in and out of their vehicles ... or walking across a parking lot. Obese folks find that normal activities such as these are often things to be dreaded. Getting out of a chair isn't something the average person thinks about ... for the bigger cohort it can be a valid fear. After all, sitting down is generally not bad, since gravity takes over on the way down ... but getting out of the chair can be a real challenge. Heck, even just the simple act of stepping off a curb is fraught with danger for many overweight people, who fear that their leg will buckle. It is understandable when faced with all the hurdles, many (particularly the morbidly obese) prefer to just stay home. By decreasing body weight while increasing workouts in a controlled fashion, many of these fears will disappear.

The Stool of Fitness

As you are no doubt aware, there are endless ways to approach physical activity. Everyone has their own ideas on how to increase your physical health, including a myriad of exercises, theories, systems, etc. As for me, I prefer to temper all things in life from the perspective of *balance* (as you will certainly notice in the Wellness section to follow!). When we begin to think about fitness, I recall somewhere in my dark past that someone characterized fitness as being like a three legged stool. The analogy was meant to show that each leg of a stool must be the same length to be balanced, so consequently your fitness would be best achieved by a similar balanced approach. How true.

I remember one such "stool" that had the three components of aerobic training, strength training, and flexibility … this is certainly a valid approach. While I believe we can follow the same basic premise here, I want to make a slight change to our stool. For the benefit of this book's target audience, I prefer to consider the three legs of our fitness stool as being *diet, aerobic training*, and *strength training*. Please don't think that I have anything against flexibility, since it is a vital component of a fit person. You should attempt to stretch and maintain your flexibility as much as you can tolerate it. Yet, as important as flexibility may be, it falls far behind the initial needs of the obese to master their diet, increase aerobic fitness, and gain physical strength. Of course, we have already covered the first leg of the stool (diet) pretty well in Chapter 4. That leaves us with aerobic training and strength training, which we will address in the next two sections. Just to remind you ... your health and fitness (and in fact your whole life) must maintain the proper balance, or else you risk ... ummm, falling off of your stool.

6.   AEROBIC TRAINING

Before you read any further, please pause for just a moment. Concentrate on your heart; more specifically, your heartbeat. Feel it thumping away in there? It's certainly no secret that your heart beats thousands and thousands of times each day. It is also a fact that the heart is part of the cardiovascular system, which functions to furnish your body with oxygen and nutrients that are needed for the body to do work. The heart is the pumping mechanism providing the motive force that moves the oxygen and nutrient filled blood around to do its job. Since the heart is a muscle itself, it adapts (along with the entire cardiovascular system) by becoming stronger and more efficient when it is placed under progressive loads. The best way to place the cardiovascular system under load is to subject it to *aerobic training*.

I'm sure you all have some clue as to the meaning of the term "aerobic." At its very basic level, aerobic means "in the presence of oxygen." Yet people who go to an "aerobics" class don't go to be in the presence of oxygen ... they go to train their cardiovascular system in an attempt to increase its aerobic fitness. Whether you refer to it as your aerobic fitness, cardio-respiratory endurance, aerobic power, cardiovascular endurance, or any other such terminology, they all allude to the capacity of the various body parts (inc. heart, lungs, blood vessels, etc.) to carry and deliver oxygen to the body to produce energy.

For our sake, maybe we can simplify it further by thinking of aerobic training as activity that increases our breathing and heart rate. A great analogy might be that of your car. If you want your car to go faster, you press the accelerator pedal more, since the engine needs more fuel to comply. Not much different with your body, since as you ask it to do more work, it too needs more fuel. Because the cardiovascular system supplies the fuel, it has to ramp up output to keep up with changing demand. The efficiency with which it does this is loosely your aerobic fitness level.

Aerobic Info (General)

As long as we're using automobile analogies … imagine you're driving along on a beautiful sunny day. You come over a small hill, and on the other side you see a police car with his radar device pointing at you. What is the first thing you do? Inevitably you will immediately glance down at your speedometer to see how fast you're going! With that in mind, wouldn't it would be pretty sweet if you had a speedometer for your body so that you could determine how hard you are working out? I'm here to report that you are in luck, since you already have that option … even better, it came as part of *your* original equipment … it's your heart!

Before we go too far, this is a good time to quickly revisit our heart … the thing we felt thumping in our chests a few paragraphs ago. Since the heart works by beating (actually contracting) to pump blood through itself and out to the body, one way to measure the work being performed by the heart is to simply count the number of times it beats in a minute. This is referred to as your pulse, or *heart rate*. The harder the heart works, the more times it needs to beat. Is heart rate the only way to determine your work load? Of course not. However, for us and our application in this book, it is perfect. Before you begin a workout plan, it is important to understand that your heart rate is a valuable tool for you to use to monitor your workouts and control their results ... both for increased aerobic fitness as well as for your safety.

There are several methods used to actually measure heart rate. First, nearly every piece of cardio equipment sold for gym or home use today has some form of heart rate monitor included, so you can hold the pads, wrap the band, attach the clip, or whatever else you need to do to have your heart rate display on the machine. There are also any number of personal devices, including strap on monitors, phone apps, etc. that you can use. In case you want to do it the old fashioned way, simply take two fingers and press them on the underside of your arm on the thumb side of your wrist. When you feel your heart beating, count the number of beats in 15 seconds, then multiply this number by 4 to calculate your total beats per minute. Or you could count for 30 seconds then multiply by two ... or you could count the beats for a full minute. Okay, you get the picture ... just count. With this proficiency, you have a method to track the effectiveness of your workout ... again, it can provide feedback to you just like the speedometer in your car does.

Now I'm sure you're thankful for the short lesson on auto mechanics being integrated with anatomy and physiology, but I bet you're also wondering what to do with this heart rate number once you can determine it. Simple ... you can use your heart rate as a guideline to measure your work load. More specifically, you will need to compare your heart rate at any time with your *maximum heart rate* (MHR).

To determine your MHR, simply subtract your age from the number 220. For instance, a healthy, fit 40 year old person will have an MHR of 180 beats per minute (220 - 40 = 180). So if our fictional 40 year old was monitoring his / her heart rate, they would know that they should never go beyond 180 beats per minute, which represents 100 percent of their MHR. You can glance at Table 6.1 below and see that we have compiled a small table that lists some ages and their corresponding MHR. Obviously if your age lies between the ones listed, your MHR will be slightly different, so take that into account.

AGE (Yrs)	Max Heart Rate (MHR)
20	200
30	190
40	180
50	170
60	160
70	150
80	140

Table 6.1 *Age and MHR Table*

Back to the vehicle comparisons for a second … if you look at the gauges in your car's dash, your speedometer gauge has a zero at one end, and a much higher number (say 120) at the other end. Does this mean you will only maintain either a speed of 0 or 120 while you drive? Of course not ... the majority of time your speed falls somewhere between those extremes. Think of your heart rate as being the same. You have a resting heart rate (say 60 beats per minute), and you can determine your MHR which sets the other extreme.

For aerobic training purposes, it is normal to try express your goals in terms of *percent of MHR*. In the table below (Table 6.2) you will note that we have expanded on Table 6.1 by adding various percentages of MHR per age. This allows you to not only determine the correct MHR, but also to determine other target heart rates as well, making it easier to find the appropriate percent of MHR to use as your goal. This is a valid and reliable tool to assist you in safely strengthening your aerobic capacity.

AGE (Yrs)	Max Heart Rate (MHR)	50% of MHR (in Beats Per Minute)	60% of MHR (in Beats Per Minute)	70% of MHR (in Beats Per Minute)	80% of MHR (in Beats Per Minute)	90% of MHR (in Beats Per Minute)
20	200	100	120	140	160	180
30	190	95	114	133	152	171
40	180	90	108	126	144	162
50	170	85	102	119	136	153
60	160	80	96	112	128	144
70	150	75	90	105	120	135
80	140	70	84	98	112	126

TABLE 6.2 *Age, MHR, and % of MHR Table*

How can this table help you? It's pretty self explanatory, but as a quick example, we'll assume we have a 60 year old man who wants to work at 70 percent of his MHR. First, we find that his MHR is 160 beats per minute. Next, we see that 70 percent of 160 equals 112 beats per minute. Therefore, our gentleman in this example will strive to increase his activity until his heart rate rises to 112 beats per minute … and he will stay as close to that number as possible for some determined length of time.

Speaking of time, the American Heart Association (AHA) recommends *moderate* exercise for at least 150 minutes per week, so that is a good goal to shoot for. What is regarded as "moderate"? Using your heart rate (or Table 6.2 if you prefer) as a guide, activity is considered moderate at 50 to 70 percent of your MHR. (Besides doing the calculation, an easy way to know if you are working at a moderate intensity is that you will feel an increase in your breathing rate, but you shouldn't be so short of breath that you can't have a conversation. In contrast, vigorous intensity causes heavy and rapid breathing, with no way to talk unless you pause for some breath every few words.) As for the 150 minutes per week suggested time requirement, think of it like eating a steak … one bite at a time! You can choose to split your 150 minutes up in almost any combination of segments, but a simple way to rationalize it is that you should be active for 30 minutes a day, five times a week. Note that this is a *minimum requirement*, and it is certainly great if you can increase this number. Even better is to plan to include some activity at least once every day. It is also important to know that the time block (for instance, 30 minutes) does not have to be consecutive … several 10 or 15 minute segments will produce results too. As the cardiovascular system adapts, it is normal to workout at a higher percentage of your MHR to see additional results. After beginning at a lower MHR to acclimate your body, you will gradually progress toward working at 50 to 70 percent of your MHR (moderate intensity), and then advance to working in the range of 70 to 85 percent of MHR (vigorous intensity) as your fitness permits.

Aerobic Training ... It Works

As you read over the information in the previous paragraphs, you may have thought that all this aerobic stuff seems a little daunting. All those numbers ... yuck. Do you remember wondering why you had to take math in school, since you just *knew* you would never use it again? Hahahaha ... well, this stuff is real world data for a real world application ... your health. You're reading this book hoping to find something that works. You have made a choice to regain control of your life through weight loss, workouts, and wellness. Hopefully you will get your eating under control, and begin to feel better. It is time to continue your progress toward wellness by incorporating workouts ... beginning with aerobic training. Why aerobic first? Frankly, because it uses the most energy in the least amount of time ... as our business and economics friends would say, it has a higher cost-to-benefit ratio.

The prime way to get the heart rate up is by walking. Other than a comfortable pair of shoes, walking doesn't require any special equipment or skill sets. A walk can increase heart rate, build stamina / endurance, strengthen muscles and tendons, and have an effect on emotional and social wellness as well. A person can vary their speed, distance, terrain, etc. to achieve and maintain their target heart rate. There are many, many places where you can safely walk, including your neighborhood, local parks, trails, and shopping malls. Oh, and in some ways walking actually has more benefits to the heavier person, since people burn more calories the heavier they are!

If instead of walking outside you choose to use your own aerobic equipment, or prefer to work out in a gym, you can reach and maintain your target heart rate by adjusting the speed, incline, resistance, or other variables on the machines. I feel that particularly in the early phase of your quest to change your body, your workouts should be regular and structured. Some exercise gurus call this *intentional training*, and that term makes sense. We could think of it as training for training sake. By performing exercises that allow you to closely monitor your physical condition and heart rate, you have a greater control over the stresses you place on your body. Yessss, I understand that mowing the grass also burns calories and increases heart rate, and please don't think I mean that you should have an overgrown yard! Feel free to do those types of things too. In fact, strive to move as much as is realistically possible based on your body's response and limitations. However, schedule your intentional training and follow through with that ... come hell or high water.

For the morbidly obese and long term sedentary, it may be that they are not initially ready to handle the extra effort of walking. They may experience back or joint pain that make walking a non-option. For them, it is necessary to find non-weight bearing exercises to do until their body adapts. A good alternative might be aquatic exercise. Water takes away much of the effect of gravity (as much as 90 percent), so exercising in water allows someone to move without as much strain. Whether you swim, or prefer aerobics, walking, boxing, or nearly any other activity, the buoyancy of water makes it easier. As your body adapts, you may consider mixing the workouts, doing aqua aerobics one day, walking on others, using aerobic equipment on another. Regardless, you have to move. Push the body and get the heart beating.

Another wonderful way to achieve your aerobic fitness goals is to do something you may not have done since you were a child ... riding a bicycle! Whether you prefer to ride an upright or recumbent stationary bike, or ride a traditional bicycle outdoors, you can receive considerable aerobic training from bikes. You can buy your own exercise bike, or know that every gym has a number of bikes available. Bikes are great for heavier folks, since they allow exercise while removing much of the weight bearing stress on the body. If you choose a traditional bicycle, that would entail a few more constraints. Most notably, you'll need a bike! Also, be sure to purchase (and wear) all appropriate safety gear. You will need to determine a safe place to ride ... while I understand that bikes have the right to be in the roadways, personally I choose to avoid riding in traffic at all costs. I have friends who are quick to point out that cars "have to recognize that your bike is the same as a car." I'm sure car drivers would be glad to respect someone on a bike ... if it wasn't for cell phones, screaming backseat kids, cell phones, automobile makeup application, cell phones, eating in the car, cell phones, self hairstyling in the vehicle … and cell phones. It only takes one mistake by a person in a car to yield catastrophic results, so I prefer not to put myself in those situations. In addition, if you don't feel your balance is good enough to ride a bicycle, investigate a tricycle, since they are more stable.

Before you race out and purchase a bike (or trike), do some research first and identify bikes that are sturdy enough for big folks. I can assure you that many of the lower end bike models you find at the local discount mart may be fine for a 13 year old who weighs as much as a sack of feathers, but for an overweight person these bikes aren't realistic. Most of the major manufacturers have at least one style / line of bikes that are sturdily built. If at all possible, go to your local bike shop and talk to the folks there, since they are knowledgeable … many times they will also have good used bikes for sale that meet your requirements. You can also certainly keep an eye on the used equipment classifieds … but the important thing is to do your research ahead of time so that you are informed.

I enjoy a bike ride in the fresh air, since it is invigorating and is generally easier on the body than the more ballistic movements. In fact, years ago when I made my commitment to increase my wellness, I would ride my bike whenever I could, even if only for a few quick trips around the block. On the weekends I would load my bike in the back of my truck and drive to various locations for an early morning ride. It is very invigorating to be riding your bike in the early morning air while watching the sun rise. I have enjoyed rides in a wide variety of locations, including through gorgeous wooded trails, beside the crashing ocean waves, along quiet rivers, and … in a local shopping mall parking lot! The mall worked out well, since there was virtually no traffic at that time of day, and the distance around the parking lot was a little over a mile … I started by doing a couple of miles, then gradually worked up as time went on. Today, many communities are putting a priority on creating / expanding bike and walking trails, recognizing that combining nature with exercise is a wonderful way to help your aerobic fitness. Regardless of the method or location you choose, it is imperative … nope, make that *mandatory* … that you begin some form of activity that will raise your heart rate and positively affect your physical wellness.

Start Your Aerobic Engine

You have done a lot of reading up to this point (I hope!), so it's time that we unveil your aerobic training plan. If you didn't know the basics of aerobic conditioning before you read this far, you certainly have a better idea by now. You know that your cardiovascular system is the major mover of blood and nutrients, and that it adapts if placed under load. You also know that your heart rate is a good indicator of workload ... and you can determine your own heart rate. Based on calculations, you can deduce your MHR, and understand that you will often work at a percentage of this MHR while doing aerobic training.

Before we launch into specific details regarding your aerobic program, we need to at least touch on the subject of how often to work out, how much to do, and how long to do it ... also known as *frequency, intensity,* and *duration*. Not to beat this to pieces, but you will be manipulating these variables for the rest of your life as you continually change your workouts to maximize their affect.

So, based on our earlier discussions, and barring any restrictions, you will use the aerobic exercise(s) of your choice in each of the three following phases. In fact, you may decide to alternate exercises, or you may choose to use several different exercises in one workout. Regardless, pay attention to the variables of frequency, intensity, and duration, while keeping in mind your heart rate as a boundary. As your health increases and your body responds, you may only be able to increase one of the variables at a time ... and that is fine. As you reach the higher limit of all three variables, ease into the next phase.

Below, I have developed 3 *Phases of Aerobic Training*, with Phase 1 for beginners, Phase 2 as a transition from beginner to a basic aerobic fitness level, and Phase 3 for those that have acquired the aerobic strength to work out at higher frequency, intensity, and duration.

Phase 1:

Frequency: 3 days per week

Intensity: Heart rate of 40 - 50 percent of MHR

Duration: Maintain elevated heart rate for 20 minutes

Note: This is generally an introductory phase, so progress as soon as possible ... maintain this phase until you can tolerate an increase in frequency, and / or intensity, and / or duration. Remember, the AHA recommends a *minimum* of 150 minutes per week at a moderate level, while this program only represents 60 minutes a week at a sub-moderate level. So you have a way to go ... get busy!

Phase 2:

Frequency: 3 - 5 days per week

Intensity:	Heart rate of 50 - 70 percent of MHR
Duration:	Maintain elevated heart rate for 20 - 40 minutes
Note:	As you enter and continue through this phase, you should concentrate on increasing frequency, intensity, and / or duration of exercise. This is where you are laying the groundwork for your future health … you will push your body to new levels here. Simple, but not always easy.

Phase 3:

Frequency:	5 - 7 days per week
Intensity:	Heart rate of 70 - 85 percent of MHR
Duration:	Maintain elevated heart rate for 40 - 60 minutes (more if you can do it)
Note:	At this level, you should have a good feel for your body and its response. You may want to investigate a variety of methods to continue challenging yourself, such as interval training, etc.

By the way, what if you can't reach the full 20 minutes in the initial phase? That just means you're a loser … a miserable failure … doomed to be an inadequate nobody for the rest of your life. You know I'm only kidding. It is not only possible, but *probable* that a good number of folks who start this plan will not be able to reach our initial goal of 20 minutes. After all, depending on who we're talking to, some folks get winded walking out to the mailbox and back ... 20 minutes of training is out of the question. While we can't possibly design individual workouts for each person in this format, one thing that we can do is to tell you ... DO WHAT YOU CAN. If 20 minutes leaves you out of gas, don't fret. Start with 3 minutes, twice a day. Or 5 minutes, 3 times a week. Whatever you can accomplish, get the heart rate up for some extended period of time. You will get benefits from this too. Just think about moving forward in the frequency, intensity, and duration of your chosen exercises. I'm positive you've heard the adage "Rome wasn't built in a day," reinforcing that the great Roman Empire was a long term, dynamic project. Think of your body as the same sort of project ... it takes time to create a polished product.

A final word here about your exercise comfort level. There is no doubt that taking your body to places it isn't used to going is certainly outside of the "comfort zone." By its very nature, exercise is meant to push the body. No matter what activity you perform to increase your heart rate, try to remember not to "fight" the movement. Don't be tense the entire time ... relax and go with it. I see people almost battling the equipment while working on an elliptical machine or treadmill ... they should loosen up. Another thing ... don't hold onto aerobic machine handles if at all possible ... you will burn more calories and increase the positive impact of the exercise by not grabbing on.

As it pertains to aerobic fitness, you know that progress is noted by the body's response to exercise as measured by heart rate. However, it is essential that you don't try to attain your long term health goals in one session! If you are exercising and your heart rate starts to creep above your target rate, slow down and allow it to recover. At this phase of your wellness journey, you are interested in increasing your aerobic fitness while burning a little fat. It is important that you recall that small steps lead to bigger ones. Be pleased with what you accomplish.

Personally ...

Something that helps me to think about my walking is to use a *pedometer*. Pedometers track how many steps you take in a day. I keep one in my pocket everywhere I go. There are about a million varieties of pedometers, but I prefer one that is about the size of a disposable lighter that I can just toss in my pocket. There is a general rule that you should try to take 10,000 steps each day, which equates to about 5 miles. Some days I make it, others I don't. Much more common is for me to be between 6,000 – 7,500 steps. The funny thing is, when I carry my pedometer, I find myself trying to add in extra steps during the day to bump up the total ... kind of a mental game. For instance, I notice I park further away from the store, or I take the garbage can and the recycle can to the street in different trips just to add another 100 steps! Hahaha, sounds crazy but it adds up. It might work for you too. One more tidbit ... if you lose your pedometer, check between the couch cushions. Yes, I've found mine there more than once.

7.   STRENGTH TRAINING

From a physiological perspective, *strength training* refers to the use of resistance exercise to cause the muscles to contract, building strength and endurance. That seems pretty simple. Ahhh, but leave it to us humans to overcomplicate the whole thing. By this time in our human existence, we have analyzed the human body *ad nauseam*. Yet, despite all the research and page after page of accumulated knowledge, we still can't even agree on how many muscles there actually *are* in the body! (Umm, before you ask, between 640 and 850). While there is no doubt that the topic of strength training can be intimidating, I beg you not try to over-think the subject. For sake of clarity, let's dig just a little bit further.

First, why should you be concerned with strength training for your body? There are a myriad of answers to that question, and I'll supply a few of the most important ones for you. First, increasing your strength will create lean muscles, leading to a better overall body composition. One positive from a leaner body is that since muscle is denser than fat, a pound of muscle takes up less space than a pound of fat ... which all means you'll be smaller. Also, strength training bolsters the various complexes (including the muscles, bones, and ligaments) that support areas such as the ankles, knees, and hips, which are notorious for being problematic for obese folks. Yet another benefit is that by increasing the amount of muscle on your body, your metabolism must work harder to support itself … this means that you are burning more calories, even after your workout is over and when sitting around or sleeping. Resistance training will also result in better bone density, which is especially important for women. You can use resistance to rehabilitate a body part that is recovering from some sort of trauma. You might even feel better in your clothes … or without them for that matter! As you will learn in the Wellness section, physical wellness affects your entire being. Okay, let's agree … strength training is good for you.

Push and Pull

Close your curtains … lock the doors. Our relationship has reached a critical point. I feel that I can trust you with some pretty significant information. The time has come for me to pass along everything you will really need to know about how to properly train your body for increased strength. Here it is … the groundbreaking information you've waited for … representing years of research … you must remember … that your body … *pushes or pulls*. That's it, case closed. It's over, done, finished, concluded, terminated. Hope you aren't too disappointed. Some people will say the body also squats, some will say it lunges, and others have their ideas too. I say hogwash … push and pull.

Think of the body as a sort of robotic machine designed to push or pull … nothing more, nothing less. At most gyms, you can find people laboring on any number of machines trying to segregate all the small muscles … in fact, they are doing very little. There is no such thing as "spot training." In a clear case of "you can't see the forest for the trees", they get so involved in trying to find exercises that address each muscle that they lose sight of our original purpose of strengthening the body. Do you recall the earlier example I gave of the days I worked in the hay fields? I can assure you that when I was lifting the hay bales to the back of a truck, I wasn't concerned whether I was isolating my rhomboid muscles from my trapezius muscles … I was just concerned with picking up all those freakin' bales! Most really heavy folks have been partially or primarily sedentary for some time, so they really shouldn't worry whether *five sets of 5 reps* is superior to a *pyramid structured* program ... they simply need to concentrate on increasing their strength through resistance training. At some time in the future, your training may progress enough that you enter a bodybuilding or fitness contest, or you may participate in a power lifting competition, or decide to compete in the local Highland Games. If so, send me an invitation ... and a ticket. But for now ... push and pull ... don't make it more than it is.

Language Requirement

Before we go any further with our section on strength training, it will be necessary for you to learn a second language. Well, not an entire language ... just *some* of the words (sorta like learning all the <u>dirty</u> words in a foreign language!). Like any subject or hobby, the strength game has its own lingo. As you progress in your strength training, you will undoubtedly be exposed to a lot of new terminology. You may know some of the terms already, or you may not. Below you will find a few of the most common terms that are used in a strength training atmosphere:

- *Compound Exercise* – multi joint movements that involve the use of more than one major muscle group ... great for building strength
- *Isolation Exercise* – single joint movements in which only one muscle group is trained
- *Rep* – short for repetition; one complete movement of one exercise from start to finish
- *Set* – consists of a certain number reps
- *Sets x Reps* – a common way to list the requirements for a particular exercise in your workout. For instance, if you are supposed to do *Pushups 3 x 12*, in English that means you will perform pushups for 3 sets of 12 reps, or 36 total pushups.

Strength Training Methods

Since I've given you the biggest secret to weight training (push and pull), we should probably discuss what methods you might to use to make your body stronger. As you can imagine, resistance can be provided in a number of ways. Common ways for folks to engage in resistance work include the use of body weight, resistance / exercise bands, weight machines, or barbells / dumbbells. Actually, you can use cans of soup, cement blocks, and old tires too ... the body doesn't care which method you use, it only knows it has to adapt to resistance.

Regarding bodyweight training, the good news is that you don't need special equipment, since you carry your workout equipment with you at all times! The exercises are familiar ... after all, anybody knows things like pushups, pull ups, free squats, lunges, and so on. Training with your body weight sounds perfect. Umm, except ... I find that the bigger people among us usually have a lot of problems with body weight exercises, mainly because they have ... so much body weight! Doing "body weight" work is usually prohibitive for bigger people, since it requires folks to work with weight that is much too heavy to accomplish many reps. No doubt that weighing more than a marshmallow brings some issues with it, including lessened flexibility and balance. Also, the act of positioning a big body for body weight exercise is usually an issue ... for instance, getting down to the floor and back up again is often too difficult to accomplish. In my experience, body weight work is useful, but is better considered after the body has achieved a little higher level of strength and flexibility ... if at all. My recommendation is that if you have other options, avoid body weight work until you have developed a base of strength to be able to do it safely and competently.

Depending on relative fitness levels, many overweight and obese people begin to strengthen their bodies using resistance bands (also known as exercise bands) at home. Resistance bands are *great* for resistance training, particularly for beginners. There are many types of bands, but primarily they are stretchy rubber / latex tubes ... a set will usually contain 4 or 5 bands, each approximately 48 inches long that can be attached to a handle. Your workout with resistance bands is only limited by your imagination ... remember that the body pushes and pulls, so use the bands to engage all the major muscle groups. Hook the bands to a chair... hang them from stair banisters ... stand on one end or in the middle ... resistance bands allow you to make some great strides toward increasing the strength and endurance of the muscles in the entire body.

Another wonderful way for those who are beginning a program or for those trying to achieve some moderate level of strength is the weight machine ... in particular the selector weight stack machines. These machines are usually fairly accessible for the bigger person to get into and out of, and they also provide a solid base, back support, and very little impact on joints. It is very easy to change the working weight on these machines, since they allow the weight to be selected by moving a pin or throwing a lever … and with no bar to balance, these machines are very safe. Big folks can perform a lot of reps in a short time on a machine, which is great for building a strength base (and good for self confidence as well). Cable machines are perfect for circuit training (more on this in a few paragraphs), which increases strength and provides aerobic training as an added benefit. Probably the only negative is that machines by their nature are designed along a fixed path of movement, which means that if you happen to be taller, shorter, wider, or more narrow than the arc of the machine, your body is often at an angle that may not be perfect. Naturally, this *may* put you at a greater chance of injury. However, since our primary goal here is to drop body weight and strengthen the body, the increase in safety as well as the convenience offered by machines gives them a lot of bonus points. Of course, to get a nice variety of machines, it generally means you have to join a gym / health club of some sort (just one of the reasons I suggest gym memberships). However, it isn't *mandatory* to use machines.

Finally, there are always the old standbys … the dumbbell and barbell (also known as free weights). As a general statement, there is nothing better in the strength training sphere than grabbing a dumbbell or barbell and going to work. They provide you with immediate feedback, since there are no adjustments …

you either move the weight … or you don't! As a big proponent of compound exercises, I can tell you that free weights force you to use many muscles to move a bar through a range of motion and back to the start. For instance, you may be able to sit in a weight machine and perform a chest press with some amount … say 135 pounds. Usually all you need to do there is adjust the seat and push the attached bar. Make no mistake, this is great and builds a nice level of strength. Yet, if you were to lie down on a standard bench to try a bench press with the same 135 pounds of free weight, you would quickly find out that the balance and stability needed to press a free bar is vastly different than the effort used in a machine. In fact, you would most likely be pretty embarrassed! So, with free weights, you are essentially doing more work than you realize. However, many of the free weight exercises need some education / training to perform them properly (which really means teaching you to get the best results without getting injured). Regardless, there is no substitute for free weights to add strength to the body … doing sets of compound free weight movements will make your whole body strong. As a beginner, particularly if you are obese, you may feel better about starting with resistance bands or cable machines until you increase your strength. However, if you choose, feel free to incorporate free weights for total body strength.

While I have supplied several methods for your use in strength training, it is not important which method you use. You can use a single method, or combine movements from all of them. Far more important than which method you use is that you actually DO use them ... train your body. Remember, use resistance to push and pull regularly, since those are the key components to gaining endurance and strength for your muscles.

Beginning Your Strength Program

First things first ... either right after you opened this book ... or before you started your new weight loss plan by changing your diet ... or before you started your workout plan by committing to increasing your aerobic training ... you should have hooked up with your doctor for a checkup. If for any reason you haven't done that by now ... shame on you! As you continue to transform your body by adding strength training, it is vital for you to know that you are medically ready to go. Strength training puts a variety of stresses on your body, and it would be smart to get a blessing from your doc. Many large guys and gals enjoy strength training, and even sedentary big people are actually stronger than they think. Makes a little bit of sense, since muscles are forced to work harder against resistance, and overweight folks do everything with lots of pounds of ... ummm, "resistance" plastered on them. Go see your primary care provider to make sure that all of the changes you are making (and hope to make) aren't harmful. Know this, all you "bigger than you want to be's" out there ... taking your body from where it is now to where you want it to be is hard work ... you should understand that the journey will be simple, but not easy. Get over yourself ... go get a checkup for your own well being.

Fresh from yet another tongue lashing about seeing a doctor ... you know that as the subtitle of this book indicates, our target audience is particularly the overweight and obese out there.

116

Of course, that may mean someone who is 25 pounds over their ideal weight, or it may be someone who is 325 pounds over theirs. There lies the problem in trying to design a comprehensive strength training plan for our readers. We dealt with this wide array of bodies and fitness levels in the aerobics section by using the heartbeat as a constant measuring stick ... there is no such commonality in strength training. You should understand that everyone (including the overweight and obese) has had different experiences when it comes to strength training.

Some may have had no exposure at all, others may have taken a weightlifting class in school, while others may have been athletes in a structured weight training program. Some may not have trained since high school, others may be gym regulars today. In an attempt to address this, we will suggest a basic program ... no, even *simpler* than basic. Our first program will be designed for those truly overweight, obese and morbidly obese, the long time overweight, and the overweight sedentaries among us. Their problem is not as complex as deciding on which sets, reps, and exercises to perform ... their problem is the act of sitting down into a chair, then standing up again. When they enter a room that has a soft, cushy couch, their hearts run cold ... they worry that if they have to sit on the couch, they may not be able to get up again. What about the effort big folks need to get in and out of their cars? Think about it ... they might be able to just open the car door, back their caboose up to the door, and fall into the car. Of course, there is also the advanced method where they attempt a semi-gymnastic ingress maneuver of putting one leg in first, then hopping sideways on the other leg in an attempt to reach the seat … praying that they have achieved the precise angle of entry … while not bashing their head against top of the doorway. Getting out can be even worse … the hip and leg strength needed to exit the vehicle is almost Olympian! Walking, navigating stairs, stepping up and down, moving on and off of a curb … all these things that many others may take for granted are real hurdles for the larger group. By following a strength training plan, our readers will strengthen their muscles that have likely not been used much for years.

The best news is that they will only need a few workouts to see huge gains … okay, that's not true … just checking to see if you were awake. Just like the other lifestyle changes we outline in this book, kick-starting a strength plan is simple, but not easy. My apologies if some of this material is too basic for some of you … just realize that there are those out there need the basic level of instruction and information. It won't hurt to read it … it's quick, and you might accidentally learn something! The truth is that the results of strength training are *directly proportional* to the work you put into it (that is your math terminology for today … thank me later).

Basic Workout for Beginners

In this section, we will present you with a basic but very good workout, designed to work the entire body using compound exercises, with the goal of strengthening the muscles of our "bigger than average" readers. We will take every precaution we can to safely and efficiently wake up the muscles that have often been dormant for quite a while. To ensure a good result on this program, you will need a few specialized pieces of equipment. First, you need ... a wall. That's right, a wall. I'm guessing you probably have some of those hanging around ... at least 4. Next, you'll definitely need ... a chair. Yep, a good sized, sturdy, chair. Up until now, I probably haven't cost you any money, since most folks have access to chairs and walls. However, I have one more item you will need. Go purchase yourself a set of resistance bands (also called exercise bands).

Resistance bands are long rubber / latex tubes, designed to attach at the end to handles. The best sets will have various colored bands in different resistance levels, enabling you to use one band or to put more than one band on the handles to generate more resistance. They are cheap, portable, compact, and effective. If you're not sure what they are or where you can find them, I did a Google online search on your behalf and returned over 7 million results ... they aren't hard to find. I promise the bands ... along with your wall and your chair, will give you an amazing variety of exercise possibilities, while increasing your strength and balance. On to the workout …

Since we are all aware of the challenges faced daily by the target reader of this book, our initial strength training plan will endeavor to strengthen the entire body using some resistance provided by bands. First things first … to start, you should expect to do *1 set of 12 reps, 2 days a week,* of each of the exercises below. Monitor how your body feels, and as soon as you think you are comfortable, try to progress. Remember our friends *frequency, intensity,* and *duration*? If you want to increase frequency, add another day a week. To heighten intensity … add more resistance. For more duration … add reps or sets. I suggest you only change one variable at a time, but definitely try to add to all three as time goes on. No particular "perfect" goals, but 3 or 4 sets of 12 reps, done 3 days a week is a good target.

As for using your bands, they are extremely sturdy, but give them a check for rips and tears before you begin your workout. Also, make sure your bands don't have any slack in them before you begin an exercise … they shouldn't be loose. If they are, take up the slack somehow … wrap them around your chair, or a hand or foot … or you could also scoot further away from wherever they are attached. Regardless, get rid of any slop before beginning. This is important because when using the bands, you should keep an even tension throughout the entire motion. Other than that, no special instructions needed … it comes back to push and pull! So, gather your walls … and your chair … and your bands … and prepare to get busy!

The Exercises

As you look at the fantastic list of exercises for you to perform, as well as the instructions that accompany them, know that I'll expect you to do them flawlessly ... but only after you warm up! Just like the car in your driveway, your body operates better if it has a warm up before working. It needs to get up to operating temperature, and to get all the fluids flowing. Resist the temptation to jump right in to a workout without any type of warm up ... your body will thank you ... for years to come.

A common way of warming up is with some light aerobic exercise. Since we are designing this workout to be done at home, we will assume you don't have any cardio equipment handy. Now, if you do have cardio equipment, and it isn't covered with clothes ... or dust ... or boxes ... feel free to do 5 – 10 minutes as a warm up. Otherwise ... I expect you to perform the old standard exercise from P. E. class ... the jumping jack! Yep, that's right ... the jumping jack is the one where you throw your hands up like you're being robbed, while at exactly the same time blasting your legs apart. Well that's how it's *supposed* to work. The saddest thing ever was watching a class of kids trying to do these exercises ... only about 25% of the participants could actually do them correctly. The rest looked like they were suffering through some sort of neurological event. With that disturbing mental image burned into my brain ... maybe we should reconsider your warm up. How about this ... you can still do jumping jacks as a warm up, but instead of bouncing your bigness all around the house, you can do them … in your chair! No, really … give it a chance!

- Exercise: *Chair Jumping Jacks*
- Sit close to the front edge of your chair, straight back, knees bent, feet touching the floor, hands in your lap
- Quickly extend your arms over your head, at the same time opening your legs to the sides, with your feet lightly landing on their heels
- Return to starting position

Note: At full extension your body should resemble an X. Do about 25 reps as quickly as possible while maintaining form. At the end of the 25 reps, feel your body … if you need more warm up, do more jumping jacks.

Just in case you don't like the jumping jacks, or can't do them without looking like the goofy kid in P. E., I'll give you an option. You may prefer to perform Step Ups.

- Exercise: *Step Ups*
- Use the wall or chair for balance if needed
- Put your entire right foot onto your platform, then bring your left foot up to meet your right, and stand on the platform

- Return to the starting position by stepping down with the right foot, then the left so that both feet are on the floor.
- Complete 20 steps leading with the right foot, then do another 20 steps leading with your left foot. Feel the body; if this is not enough warm up, do sets of 10 until you are ready to begin the workout.

Note: You'll need to find something to use as a platform to step up on to ... a stair is perfect, and so is a sturdy step stool ... or you can use a block of wood, a telephone directory, anything sturdy enough to hold your weight without breaking or sliding. I would shoot for something around 6 inches high.

All warm? Great ... here we go ... 1 set of 12 reps of each of the following exercises, done 2 days a week to start:

1. CHEST

- Exercise: *Chest Press*
- Sit in your chair and place the band at shoulder level behind your back or around the back of the chair
- Hold the handles in each hand with elbows bent
- Press forward until your arms are straight
- While squeezing the chest muscles, pause for a single count, then slowly return handles to the starting position

Note: The chest is worked by pushing. As you progress, you may want to add other chest exercises, such as push-ups, incline / decline presses, and flyes.

2. SHOULDERS

- Exercise: *Overhead Press* (also called military press, shoulder press)
- Sit close to the front edge of your chair, straight back, knees bent, feet flat on the floor
- Put the middle of the band under your feet
- Holding the handles with each hand, bring your hands to shoulder height, palms facing out (forward)
- Press hands straight up until arms are straight
- Pause for a single count, then slowly return handles to the starting position

Note: The shoulders are worked by pushing *and* pulling. As you progress, you may want to add other shoulder exercises such as upright rows, shrugs, front raises, lateral raises, and bent flyes.

3. BACK

- Exercise: *Seated Row*
- Sit in your chair, straight back, legs straight with heels resting on the floor
- Put the middle of the band under your feet

- Hold the handles with each hand, arms straight, palms facing each other
- Bend the elbows, pulling the handles toward the middle of your body
- Pause for a single count, then return to the starting position

Note: The back is worked by pulling. While performing rows, concentrate on driving the elbows backward. If you are doing rows with one arm, the movement will resemble starting a lawn mower with a pull cord. As you progress, you may want to add other back exercises such as lat pulldowns, bent rows, and pullovers.

4. **LEGS**

- Exercise #1: *Calf Press* (also called *calf raises*)
- Sit close to the front edge of your chair, straight back, legs straight with heels resting on the floor
- Put the middle of the band under the ball of one foot (it may be better to loop the band completely around the foot once to prevent it from sliding)
- Starting with the foot pointing toward the ceiling (or as close to straight up as possible), press the ball of the foot away from you as far as possible
- While squeezing the calf, pause for a single count, then return to the starting position

- Change feet after you finish your reps, and repeat the exercise

Note: Calves are worked by pushing. Don't neglect your calf muscles. Calves are sometimes called the "heart" of the lower body, since they not only serve to bend the foot, but also act as a pump to push blood back up to the body. For many sedentary or big folks, working the calves can greatly increase leg circulation, reduce leg swelling, and assist in increasing your weight bearing aerobic training ability. They are a dense muscle, since they are forced to work each time you take a step, so they can handle high weights and high reps. As you progress, you may want to add other calf exercises such as standing calf raises.

- Exercise #2: *Leg Press*
- Sit close to the front edge of your chair, straight back, legs straight with heels resting on the floor
- Put the middle of the band under one of your feet
- Holding the handles with each hand, bend your knee toward your body, then press the leg back to the starting position (straight out)
- Change feet after you finish your reps, and repeat the exercise

Note: As you progress, you may want to add other leg exercises such as leg extensions, leg curls, and lunges, and squats.

5. ARMS

- Exercise: *Bicep Curls*
- Sit close to the front edge of your chair, straight back, knees bent, feet flat on the floor
- Put the middle of the band under your feet
- Holding the handles with each hand, arms straight, palms facing the ceiling, curl your hands upward toward your shoulders
- At the top of the exercise, squeeze the bicep, pause for a single count, then return to the starting position

Note: Biceps are worked by pulling. As you progress, you may want to add other bicep exercises such as concentration curls and hammer curls.

- Exercise: *Tricep Overhead Extensions*
- Sit in your chair, straight back, knees bent with feet resting on the floor
- Place the band under your butt
- Holding the handles with each hand, elbows by your ears and pointing toward the ceiling, hands behind you
- Straighten the elbow and move your hands toward the ceiling until arms are straight
- Squeeze the triceps, pause for a single count, then return to the starting position

Note: Triceps are worked by pushing. As you progress, you may want to add other tricep exercises such as pressdowns, kickbacks, and close grip presses.

6. ABDOMINALS

- Exercise: *Seated Crunch*
- Wrap the band around the back of your chair, with the handles in front of your chest
- Sit in your chair, with a straight back, keeping your feet flat on the floor during the entire exercise
- While holding the handles in each hand, tighten your stomach muscles, then slowly lean forward as far as you can, pause for a single count, then return to the starting position

Note: Yes, overweight, obese, and morbidly obese people have abs too! No matter how much extra "padding" you may have, I assure you that everyone has stomach muscles. Abdominals are the muscles that support the abdomen and help keep the trunk erect. You must strengthen your abdominal section so that it can function properly. Oh, I'm sure some of you want to show off your hidden 6 pack … but all the concentration on abdominal work in the world will not cause these muscles to automatically pop out. You must clean up your diet and work on removing the blubber layer that covers them. Just because you don't have rippling abs to show off, don't let that stop you from performing abdominal work ... strong abdominal muscles are vital. As a general statement, lower abs respond to leg raises, obliques (the "love handles") respond to side bends, and upper abs respond to crunches. The seated crunch used here works the upper abs, while being safer for the neck and back than crunches on the floor. As you progress, you may want to add other abdominal exercises such as leg lifts, side bends, and twists.

Oh, and about using an exercise ball ... lots of trainers feel that this is a great way for large people to improve their balance and abdominal strength. While this may be factually true, I never liked the idea of exercise balls for big folks, mainly for two reasons: people worry about falling off the ball, and they also worry whether the ball can hold their weight. Although my grandsons have a blast jumping on balloons to hear them pop, that scenario wouldn't be quite as funny if it happened to an overweight person! Save the exercise balls for the future ... or forget them completely.

Bonus Exercise

There are many who feel that the squat is the "king of exercises", and although others may make a case for the deadlift, it is hard to argue that the squat is at the top. What makes the squat so special? Let's discuss that quickly.

Just a glance at someone doing a squat and you can tell it

works the leg, back and butt muscles ... and trust me, they do. However, squats are such a tough compound exercise, it causes the body to release muscle growth "stuff" ... which means that squats positively affect muscular growth and strength in the entire body, not just the legs. The ability of squats to strengthen muscles, stabilizers, and abdominals helps you to maintain your balance, prevents injuries, and burn more fat. Squats even help you with the digestive process, assisting to move waste through the body ... and squats even help you to get down to and up from the toilet when the waste ... reaches its final destination! Because of the importance I place on squatting movements, I am going to urge you to begin some form of squatting as soon as possible. I suggest you start with the following squat:

- Exercise: *Chair Squat with Balance Assist*
- Stand in front of your chair as though you were going to sit down, feet shoulder width or wider
- Anchor your band in front of you around furniture, stair banister / rails, or whatever is sturdy enough to use as a balance point for stability during the movement
- Holding the handles in each hand, release the hips first, and sit back on the chair ... do not fall into the chair, but use the leg muscles to control your movement
- Pause on the chair for a single count, then use your legs to stand and return to the starting position

Note: This is a great take off on the traditional barbell squat. It allows you to work on standing and sitting, which may be difficult for the obese. Using the chair behind you for safety, this movement strengthens all of the associated muscles, while the band provides much some needed stability. You can rely on the bands to assist you, but their function is only as a slight force booster and for stability during the exercise ... you are not to completely support the body weight using the band while moving up or down during the exercise. USE YOUR MUSCLES! As you progress, you may want to add other squat exercises, such as squatting to the chair without bands and squatting without a chair.

There you have it ... a basic, no frills, beginner type workout. It is designed to be done at home, using a wall ... and a chair ... and some resistance bands. Up to this point, my suggestion has been to get your eating plan under control, then begin your aerobic conditioning. With those accomplished, it is time to move on with this strength training. Everything you need is here ... you just have to plug yourself into the equation and start working.

While designing this workout, it was important to consider all the variables. First, with our target reader in mind, the choice of using resistance bands for our example was fairly easy. Bands are cheap, compact, portable ... and available. They require no special training, and can be used at home, on a trip, or even at work if you're the boss! Bands don't lock your body into one motion, and can be used in a variety of movements. In short … they work. You may choose to stay with resistance bands from now on. That is nothing to sneeze at, since the benefits offered by the bands are many.

If you do choose to go to a gym, whether you prefer weight machines, free weights, or some combination, the goal is the same … train the whole body, preferably doing multi- joint, compound exercises. Since there is a good chance you are overweight, I would suggest that you not try to heave a lot of iron around … at least not until you reduce your body weight, increase your tolerance to workouts, advance your aerobic conditioning, and bolster your muscle strength and endurance. My program for you would contain lighter weights, more reps and sets. The plan presented here is a good example of a simple program that addresses the entire body, and is practical for our audience. As I said earlier, there is no way for us to cover all exercises for all methods in our book … especially if I want to keep it under 1,000 pages! Many of you will want to experience what machines and free weights have to offer … I understand. I hit the gym regularly myself, and along with some aerobic work, I use a combination of free weights and machines. However, always remember that no matter what format you choose to change your body's strength, it always comes back to push and pull … nothing more.

Circuit Training

One of the overall goals of increasing physical wellness for the obese is to reduce body weight by controlling the diet, while at the same time increasing the work that the body does. Generally speaking, resistance training is not a huge calorie burning event. Likewise, aerobic activities are not known for their muscle building qualities. For our purposes, wouldn't a combination of the two provide better results? Good question ... the answer is *yes it would*. And it has a name ... *circuit training*.

Circuit training is a workout that is structured in a way that you will perform a series of strength training exercises back to back ... with the difference being that you will take no breaks except when moving from exercise to the next. A circuit can easily be done using any method, including with your body weight, rocks, milk jugs, resistance bands, free weights, machines ... you get the picture. You can also use any or all of these in combination to circuit train. Since you work with higher repetitions and move quickly from one strength exercise to the next, you not only receive muscular benefit, you receive an aerobic workout as well. In addition, a circuit training workout will burn more calories and reduce the length of your workout.

Sounds good ... so how can you perform a circuit training workout? First, select around 10 different exercises, generally alternating between push and pull movements, or between upper and lower body movements. Perform the first exercise, then quickly move to the next, then the next, all the way through the list of exercises you chose. The key to circuit training is speed, since the only rest you take is however long it takes you to go from one station to the next … hopefully less than 30 seconds. It should be obvious that the limited rest time between exercises will function as an aerobic training generator, which when added to the strength training component, serves to work the body at a higher level. I would suggest that you may consider using circuit training after you have been training for a few months. You should maintain the exercise weight amounts so that you can just barely finish 20 reps on each exercise. Increase days of the week, weight amounts, and circuits as tolerated. This is a quick, efficient, training plan that works. It is a perfect example of a system that is simple, but not always easy.

Breathe In, Breathe Out

Oh, by the way ... while you lift weights, please breathe. Feel free ... say it ... "now you're telling us we have to breathe ... wow, no kidding, stupid ... to think I paid for that great info." Be nice ... believe it or not, there is a proper way to breathe while tossing around the pounds. It basically involves *breathing out under strain*. Holding your breath under strain can cause a rapid increase in blood pressure, and also increase the internal pressure in the abdomen, contributing to hernias. So try to practice the command of your breathing, striving to breathe out during the most strenuous portion of the exercise. For instance, in a classic bench press, you would breathe in while lowering the bar to the chest, then breathe out while pushing the bar away. While you already have enough to remember as a beginning lifter, it is important to master your breathing. Don't hold your breath ... air in, air out.

Personal Observations

As we approach the end of the strength training section, I have compiled several observations regarding strength training that I've made through the years. As an experienced writer and published author, I could have used my clever and sophisticated writing ability to weave these observations together into other parts of this chapter. I didn't … but I think they're worthy of space in this book anyway! Read on.

Observation 1 ... Perception

Perception is very important when discussing strength training. Many times while talking with folks (particularly women) about resistance training, they tell me "I honestly want to work out, but I don't want to get really big and muscular!" I could scream when I hear that! Can you imagine someone sitting down at the piano for the very first time and saying "Look, I want to play the piano, but I don't want to play as well as Tchaikovsky." That statement is just as wacky as the worry over getting too big before even picking up a weight! I have to calmly tell them that without years and years of dedication, nutrition, supplementation, the right genetics, etc. they won't magically blow up into a behemoth. These "really big and muscular" physiques that they fear belong to a small portion of the top one percent of all folks who incorporate resistance training into their workout programs. As Dan John (2015) writes, "Big, strong people eat big, sleep big, fart big, and train with huge loads on their back." Point taken ... it isn't an accident that big, muscular people get that way. Plus, for the majority of readers of this book, at this stage of your quest for health, getting "big" is actually the opposite of what you want to do ... heck, you're already big! Concentrate on making your body leaner and stronger; never fear, you won't magically wake up one day and be huge and muscle bound!

Observation 2 ... Magazine Syndrome

Unfortunately, I can't blame the average person for having the perceptions noted in Observation 1. It is just a symptom of something I call the "magazine syndrome." This common and troubling phenomenon is characterized by the opening of the mouth, followed by a diarrhea-like regurgitation of knowledge about sets, reps, exercises, secret programs, supplement stacks, drinking magic hydro replenishment fluid after every rep, this machine, that machine, and on and on. Frankly, it is very reminiscent of pulling the string on the back of a doll and listening to the same crap repeated over and over again. The source of all this erudite wisdom is usually one of the many fitness magazines that flood the market (hence the "syndrome" terminology). While I use magazines as my target, with the technology at our fingertips today the internet is as much at fault, if not more. For their part, magazines exist to make money through advertising and supplemental sales; they are a business. Please read them if you desire, since they are full of information. Just keep in mind that the information is not meant to be a comprehensive bible of strength training, so take it with the proverbial grain of salt.

Observation 3 ... Everything Old is New Again

If you have been around the strength training arena ... and you are fortunate to live long enough ... you will see truth in the statement "everything old is new again." This is a great quote, and it personifies the strength training game. Despite the fact that somebody always wants to discover a new method of training your body, there are really only so many ways to overload your muscles (recall push and pull?). As I workout, there are times when I am approached by others who will quiz me about the "old school" exercises I am doing. Of course, since I prefer to work out with iPod music blasting into my ears, my first clue of people asking me questions is when I see them standing in front of me with their lips moving! However ... I will usually try to remove the ear buds and have a quick discussion with them. More often than not, this "mysterious" exercise is nothing more than some form of compound lift that has been performed for years and years. Yes, people were doing these things BEFORE magazines and web sites! I can't fault the questioners completely, since they haven't seen that particular movement in any of their magazines (the syndrome strikes again). One younger guy who worked out with me for a short time laughed and said my workouts were like prison workouts! I took that as a complement, since he was suggesting that there was nothing flashy, only a minimum of special machines used, and plenty of hard work involved. Today, that often qualifies as outside the norm.

<u>Observation 4 ... Feeling Frustrated ... Functionally</u>

The strength training arena is no stranger to questionable fads, wacky practices, "can't miss" equipment, and ever changing terminology. One example is the fairly recent term *functional training*. Definitions vary, but generally they go something along the line of *training using movements that are specific to one's activities of daily living*. If that's true, can anyone give me an idea of exactly what "activities of daily living" require the ability to plaster butts on big rubber balls while doing dumbbell curls with 2.5 pound dumbbells? I have to confess that when I see someone using one of those balls, it reminds me of going to the circus when I was young and watching the elephants perch their big bodies on top of a ball ... I guess the pachyderms were increasing their functional abilities without knowing it. *Anyway* ... I've also heard functional exercises referred to as being *multi-muscle, multi-joint movements*. Funny, before "functional training" those movements were called ... compound exercises. And how do you train functionally for ... life? For instance, when it's time to change a tire, or to get the boxes full of Christmas decorations out of the attic, or to pull bags of groceries out of your car trunk ... it's doubtful that you have specifically trained functionally for those situations. So do you drive with a flat, skip Christmas, and have to eat out of your trunk? Probably not. It should be obvious that ANY exercise you do to strengthen your body is *functional*. The term "functional training" to me seems to be a gimmick to allow trainers (including

141

well-meaning ones) to wow clients with their abilities to mysteriously identify *exactly* those "special" exercises needed to prepare them for everyday life! Nothing special is needed ... strive to work your entire body. That will result in an overall body wellness and balance ... regardless of whatever the next fancy terminology is.

Personally ...

Because it is obvious that many ... many ... many people haven't been told the rules of gym etiquette, I am going to perform a public service for them. I'm hoping to save them from glares, harsh words, or being stuck in a trash can head first. I'm sure that they have read the rules before they signed on the bottom line at the gym ... they probably just accidentally overlooked a few areas. Because the only other explanation is that they feel that the rules are for everyone but them ... which would lead back to the ... glares, harsh words, and being stuck in a trash can head first. So, in no particular order:

- *Don't Interrupt* – the time to talk to people in the gym is not when they are in the middle of a set ... at minimum, wait until they finish their set to ask them whatever is so important it just can't wait ... for instance, *"Excuse me, but what is the name of that odd looking, old school exercise you're doing? It seems so ... functional."*

- *Clean The Equipment* – understand that I'm happy you have a good sweat going, but I'm not as excited about your perspiration as you are ... so spray and wipe the equipment when you finish using it.

- *Put Your Weights Back* – this means taking the plates off the bar, and returning them to the plate trees or designated areas ... this doesn't mean throwing them on the floor. Also, return dumbbells to the racks, and any attachments to their home location. Come on ... you put 'em on, so take 'em off.

- *No Curls In A Squat Rack* – PLEASE don't tie up a squat rack (or power rack) with your attempt to work on your bulging biceps ... you can do curls on any bench, in the corner with dumbbells, on machines, and lots of other ways, but it is very tough to do heavy squats, deadlifts, etc. without a rack.

- *Don't Circuit Train If The Gym Is Busy* – although I am a big proponent of circuit training, you must realize that the gym has other patrons beside you. It isn't realistic for you to work on, say 6 different machines while others stand around and wait. When I start to use a piece of equipment, and suddenly someone runs half a mile across the gym to tell me that they are using it, my response is the same ... "No you're not ... if you were using this, we wouldn't be having this conversation."

- *Finish Your Sets, Then Move* – don't loiter on a machine ... they really aren't designed to be used as a park bench. Do your sets ... clean the machine ... move on. I was working out one time, and a friend of mine was working out in the same section of the gym. My buddy was a pretty big, strong guy, and was normally very quiet. This particular day, he wanted to use an adjustable utility bench, but it had a towel on it … which generally means someone is using it. I watched as the towel owner would do a set elsewhere in the gym, then return to wipe himself off with the towel … which he would then put back on the bench. My friend passed by the bench a number of times, and was starting to get frustrated. Finally, my friend … and the towel owner … and the towel … all met at the bench in question … where my friend bellowed *"Is this a bench or a @&#$ing towel rack?"* I watched the towel owner grab his towel and flee … all the while I was laughing hysterically! The moral is, use common sense … the gym is for everyone … don't monopolize equipment by sitting on it forever … or by leaving your towel on it.

8.   Wellness

"The part can never be well unless the whole is well."
Plato (Greek philosopher)

Wellness Defined

The term wellness has become a common term in our daily lexicon ... it's one of those words that is often heard, sometimes used in conversation, but is rarely understood. So what is wellness, and what does it mean? It is difficult to assign an exact definition to wellness ... and to make matters worse, there really is no universal definition. Many times when you see the term wellness, it is explained as being a *state of well being*. Ummm ... nice blahhh definition, but that certainly leaves the reader lacking. Then, there is also the interpretation that is considered the medical model, stating that health / wellness are considered to be solely *an absence of disease or disability*. Of course, this is somewhat true, since at face value the absence of disease can classify as wellness ... yet, that still doesn't address the more complete wellness condition.

Possibly the most comprehensive definition that I have seen comes from the National Wellness Institute and asserts that wellness is *"an active process of becoming aware of, and making choices toward, a more successful existence"* (Wellness, 2016). What is it about this definition that sets it apart? Perhaps because it says so much while saying so little. It certainly infers that there is no discernible start and finish with wellness ... rather, wellness is to be thought of as an ongoing process that consists of small changes constantly leading toward a perceived goal. What isn't specifically noted in the above definition is the fact that wellness integrates the *entire* being, including physical, psychological, social, and spiritual components. This interactive, deliberate process requires each person to become more aware of their health through information gathering, controlling harmful risk factors, and making choices that will result in a better life balance. To truly be well, each area of life must be cultivated to achieve a healthy balance.

So, as a means of a reminder, my favorite definition of wellness is worth repeating ... "*an active process of becoming aware of, and making choices toward, a more successful existence.*" I'm not sure it could be stated any better.

Personally ...

For those of simple mind (like me), I suppose you could summarize the concept of wellness by comparing it to a big pot of grandma's beef stew. She would lovingly sear the stew meat, caramelize the onions, chop carrots and potatoes, toss in the peas, and brown the flour to make the gravy. She would combine all these things in a big pot, throw in the right amount of salt and pepper, then cook it for several hours, resulting in a wonderful amalgam of tastes. But ... what if granny got a little senile and forgot one or more of the critical ingredients? The stew would be edible, but not nearly the complex gastronomic delicacy it was before. Your wellness is the same way ... if one area is weak or missing, you will not be complete. Strive for balance in your life to achieve wellness. If you don't, you may turn out to be ... a few ingredients short of a stew! (That's a good one ... I should copyright that ...)

Wellness Through the Ages

So, how about it...when you hear the word "wellness", do you think that it must be some sort of fancy new age term for eating pine bark? Or maybe the latest in a long line of *blah blah blah* created by skinny people in Spandex? Hahaha ... au contraire, my friends. While the exact origin of the wellness concept is unknown, it is certain that it is at least 5,000 years old! Regardless of origin, widespread use of the word "wellness" was not popular until the 20th century in the United States.

As hard as it is for me, I want to be completely serious for a moment. It is vitally important for you to be exposed to the history of wellness to gain some perspective on its past, present, and future, as well as to understand how important the concept of wellness really is. For instance, if you think of how impactful our earlier chapters are, you know that they provide a path for the overweight and obese to make profound changes in their lives. Pretty significant, wouldn't you agree? So how do you feel when I tell you that *all the things we have discussed up to now are only just a small part of wellness?*

I know what you're thinking now ..."but please Bruce, anything but history!" Calm down ... you have already been exposed to new ideas and information in this book, and you've survived! As a student of history, I understand the importance of the past. However, I know that many of my readers may not have the same appreciation. Because of that, I'll give you a quote that sums up why we should examine history. It comes from German philosopher Georg Hegel, who writes *"We learn from history that man can never learn anything from history."* Ooops ... wrong quote! Here we are ...a quote from G.K. Chesterton, English writer, poet, and philosopher who noted that *"...we can be almost certain of being wrong about the future, if we are wrong about the past."* There we go ... much better! Now off we go through the ages!

Wellness in Antiquity

When trying to pinpoint the beginnings of wellness, an easy place to begin is in India with the idea of *Ayurveda*. Ayurveda means the "knowledge or science of longevity", and was a collection of medical knowledge that focused on prevention as well as treatment. Although the Ayurveda was first documented around 1500 BCE in Hindu texts, it is estimated that the knowledge was passed down orally for at least 1500 years before that!

The Chinese were also great contributors to the wellness concept. They believed that the body (and mind) was basically a highway that carried energy flow ... and that relative health was measured by the efficiency of the flow. The Chinese would develop the concept of yin-yang, illustrating that although all things have two halves, the halves are never stationary, but are always changing in an attempt to achieve and maintain balance and harmony. So if you were sick, the focus was on returning you to a balance between yin and yang. As a side note, some of their tools to achieve balance are still being employed some 3500 years later, including acupuncture, acupressure, tai chi, and herbal medicine to name a few.

Other great civilizations also were known for their theories and research regarding wellness. The ancient Greeks felt that medicine was a dynamic mix of both physical and spiritual components. They worshipped Aesculapius, the semi-mythical son of Apollo, as the god of medicine. Furthermore, Greek legend notes that Aesculapius had two daughters, Hygeia and Panacea. Hygeia is considered to be the goddess of preventative medicine, while her sister Panacea is the goddess of treatment … this paradox between prevention and treatment is still evident in the medical field today, particularly when discussing the nature of wellness.

As time passed, the impact of gods was sanctioned by fewer Greek physicians … the idea arose that people should bear much more of the accountability for disease than was previously thought. Possibly the most famous of all Greek physicians was Hippocrates, known as the Father of Modern Medicine. Hippocrates, who lived from approximately 460 BCE – 370 BCE, is generally credited with minimizing the spiritual influence on the field of medicine … his actions actually began to make medicine a logical science. He scientifically conducted experiments that proved disease was caused not by gods, but by natural reactions of the body itself. His ideas and practices are closely aligned with holistic practices of today. He felt that the body was in perfect balance when its four "humors" (phlegm, blood, yellow bile, and black bile) were balanced. If these humors were to become unbalanced, disease was the result. To rebalance the humors, natural substances were given to re-establish balance, and therefore remedy the disease. Hippocrates also recognized that disease was caused by factors such as diet, living habits, and the environment, and as such, held that prevention was as important as treatment.

The Romans followed the Greeks, and simply put, preferred to prevent disease as opposed to cure it. In contrast to the Greeks who felt that health was a private issue, the Romans felt that since public health benefitted the entire empire, the government should encourage and support measures to enhance it. While the Romans didn't necessarily understand the concept of germs, they recognized that a relationship existed between personal hygiene and disease. Since hygiene was greatly affected by water and sewage, the Romans would engineer and build an aqueduct system to bring fresh water to the populace. Also, extensive use was made of public baths and bath houses. In addition, toilets were not uncommon in Roman homes, or even in public locations. Many of these toilets operated using an advanced sewer system. It has been noted that "By 315 AD, it is said that Rome as a city had 144 public toilets which were flushed clean by running water" (Trueman, 2015). There can be no doubt that Rome's focus on public health enabled the population to remain healthier … in other words, they had increased the wellness of the people.

As we know from history, the Roman Empire would eventually fall. Of course, it wasn't exactly a "fall", but more of a "decline", so an exact date is impossible to determine. It is generally offered that when the last of the Roman Emperors

(Augustulus Romulus) was ousted in 476 CE by Germanic tribes, this is considered the end of the empire ... as well as the unofficial beginning of the *Dark Ages*. In a classic understatement, this "Dark Age" in Medieval Europe did not promote many advances in healthcare. During this time, the Catholic Church was not only the religious center, but also provided the only organized medical treatment ... monks, priests, and nuns often provided the only care for sick people. Despite their altruistic role in caring for mankind, the Church could also be accused of actually impeding medical progress, since they felt that disease was God's punishment, and as such, they forbade most medical procedures. The Dark Ages were truly dark as it related to medical advancement, and resulted in little medical / wellness advancement for approximately one thousand years.

Wellness 1400 CE – 1800 CE

In approximately the year 1400 CE, and lasting roughly 300 years, an intellectual movement began in Europe that allowed the transformation of the population from the medieval age to the modern era ... we know this movement as the *Renaissance*. The Renaissance is known for great advances in literature and the arts, as well as the beginning of modern science. One of the major changes to medicine during the Renaissance was the further development of the "scientific method" by a variety of scientists and philosophers. This new method used rational, logical steps to prove by observable facts and results ... an approach that could be best characterized as "seeing is believing." It proved a dramatic shift from the past ... and its widespread use and success would change the face of medical treatment forever.

One of the great thinkers spawned by the Renaissance was Rene' Descartes. Descartes, who oddly enough was a mathematician, surmised that the mind and body are two completely separate entities. This concept would be known as *dualism*, and proposed that because the mind and body were separate, they should be treated as such medically. This theory that a disconnect existed between mind and body was revolutionary in its own right, since up to this point in history, medical treatment had been more apt to consider an approach which treated the person as a whole. So, a new dichotomy arose where physicians began to concentrate strictly on the body, while philosophers (later psychiatrists) were consulted for anything related to the mind. Testament to its impact, this basic format of dualistic philosophy still guides patient care some 350 years after the Renaissance.

Time continued to march on, and increased concentration on treating the body spread throughout Europe. As was repeated throughout history, trends in the United States often followed those of Europe ... and so it was with medicine. In the American colonies, before the development of biomedicine, physicians often classified sickness using the same "imbalance of humors" theory championed by Hippocrates over 2,000 years earlier! With that in mind, many early medical procedures involved bloodletting (either by cutting or by using leeches) ... the presumption being that letting out blood induced sleep and reduced pain. In addition, many times the bleeding procedure was combined with medicine that would create diarrhea and vomiting, surmising that by reducing the level of bodily fluids, it would not allow the illness to survive. Notably, even the first U.S. President, George Washington, was treated using these methods. Two years after he retired from the presidency, he awoke with a throat infection, so the attending physicians bled him a number of times. It is estimated that five pints of blood were taken from him, which is half the blood volume of a normal man. The resulting weakness is said to have contributed to (or actually caused) his death, making Mr. Washington the first *ex-president* in more ways than one!

Wellness 1800 CE – 2000 CE

Combining the scientific method with the idea of dualism, medical research exploded. Biological factors became the focus, resulting in increased knowledge of diseases and how they infected humans. Scientists such as Louis Pasteur proved the existence of micro-organisms that caused sickness; of course, we know these organisms as "germs." This new "germ theory" would be immensely important for the understanding of disease, illness, and health by physicians. In the mid 1800s, the germ theory would prove to be the predecessor of the "biomedical model", which evolved to focus *strictly* on biological factors, and resulting in a premise that if the patient is free from disease or pain, they are "healthy." Note that *only biological options* were considered, failing to consider any external influence from other factors such as social or psychological stressors … a thought process which is still reflected today in Western medicine.

By the late 1800s, the United States had become a relatively prosperous country, with an economy that relied on manufacturing and industry. Economic growth occurred at unparalleled pace, resulting in an industrial strength that equaled that of European countries. During this period, even though the biomedical model was the accepted norm in the medical field, a wide variety of people chose to support (and partake in) many of the "alternative" medical practices of the day. Numerous people made major contributions to this whole body wellness movement

... one particular free spirited thinker was John Kellogg. In 1876, Kellogg became the superintendent of a small health institute in Michigan, where he used natural healing methods to teach his visitors how to get well and stay well. Kellogg called his techniques "biologic living", which he said resulted in "health, comfort, efficiency, long life. It means good digestion, sound sleep, a clear head, a placid mind, content and joy to be alive." (The Simple Life). Sort of sounds like a definition of wellness! He included a total body regimen, and felt that fresh air was vitally important, as well as climbing hills and stairs, swimming, and running. Although there was no way he could have known, Kellogg was advancing the theory of "cardio" long before it became accepted!

He also felt that a half gallon of water a day was vital, believed that proper posture was important, and regarded daily enemas as fundamental to keep intestines cleansed and thus disease free. There was to be absolutely no coffee, tea, chocolate, or cane sugar. A proponent of vegetarianism, Kellogg felt that the diet should have no meat, and very little milk, cheese, and eggs. In addition to his dietary advice, Kellogg thought that meals should be enjoyed, stating that everyone should "dismiss work, worries, business cares and annoyances while eating. Good cheer promotes good digestion. Anger, worry, irritation, stop digestion." (The Simple Life). Hmmm ... I'm thinking Kellogg wouldn't be a big supporter of racing through the drive-through window of a fast food joint on the way to his next stop! Yet, as well known as Kellogg was for his skills as a wellness promoter, surgeon, and inventor, he would be best remembered because of ... an accident!

In an attempt at cutting costs for his institute, Kellogg and his brother often invented their own foods made from various grains. One particular day, the Kellogg brothers forgot about the batch of wheat grain product they had prepared earlier ... when they found it, it seemed overcooked and dried out. Unwilling to lose an entire batch of product, the brothers decided to bake the wheat flakes to see if they would be edible. Unknown to them at the time, they had invented wheat flakes, which along with corn flakes, would become the main cereal products for a burgeoning food company ... which of course would be named Kellogg's! I would hazard a guess that their products have probably graced every table in America since then!

During the late 1800s and into the 1900s, those (like Kellogg) who chose to promote wellness instead of being a champion of the biomedical model were often considered quacks, impostors, and frauds. However, this didn't deter many from choosing to think "outside the box" when it came to health. This time period saw a number of new philosophies and methods come into being, particularly the manual therapy fields such as chiropractic, osteopathy, homeopathy, and physical therapy to name a few. Yet, well into the twentieth century, a large chasm existed between the traditional medical field and the holistic camp. In 1948, an interesting approach was taken by newly formed World Health Organization (WHO). The WHO, an agency of the United Nations, offered a definition of the word *health*, considering health to be "a state of complete physical, mental and social well-being and not merely the absence of disease or infirmity" (WHO definition of Health). It is noteworthy that this definition is one of the first to suggest that health may be more than just "not being sick" ... rather, that it was a whole person condition. In fact, it actually loosely described what would later become better known as wellness.

Despite the new notions, the "drugs and surgery" approach of the conventional medical community was still the treatment path most accepted by the American public during this period. Sadly, at times the give and take between the two divergent approaches resembled two children arguing over whether "my daddy can beat up your daddy." In 1960s, the American Medical Association (AMA) did all that it could to discredit chiropractors, going so far as to create a *Committee on Quackery* in 1963 with the goal of eliminating chiropractic. They went so far as to state that the "Committee's primary goal was to contain and eliminate chiropractic" (Chiropractic Antitrust Suit). Wow...don't hold back! This logic pretty much summed up the chasm between traditional medicine and alternative medicine. (As a side note, the law would eventually provide some relief to chiropractors in 1987 when the AMA was found guilty of defaming non-traditional physicians, distributing propaganda, refusing collaboration, and denying hospital access ... in short, they were found to be seeking a healthcare monopoly.)

In this contentious atmosphere, development of the total wellness philosophy would continue to move forward in the 1970s. Dr. John Travis would have a major impact, including his creation of the *Illness - Wellness Continuum*, a graph that follows the WHO definition of health by showing that wellness isn't only lack of disease, but should also use the variables of mental and emotional health to determine wellness. Author Don Ardell was also instrumental, penning the book *High Level Wellness*. He noted that the term wellness "has gotten confused with holistic health, disease prevention, health education and health promotion. Somehow wellness got 'stuck' in the health field, which has more of a disease/treatment framework" (Monroe, 2006). He also felt that it's "often easier for people to think of wellness in terms of 'quality existence' rather than health" (Monroe, 2006). Ardell is a firm believer in the individual's impact on their own health, exhibited by the classic statement "A consequence of this focus is that a wellness mind set will protect you against temptations to blame someone else, make excuses, shirk accountability, whine or wet your pants in the face of adversity" (Ardell, 2000). Hahaha, absolute perfection! Another of the important contributors to the idea of promoting balance and personal responsibility to achieve a healthier existence was Dr. William Hettler. In 1976, Hettler released his famous model known as the Six Dimensions of Wellness, which surmised that if people would seek an overall balance in their lives, they could bring about an increased level of well being (or "wellness"). This model and the research behind it would lead Hettler to co-found the National Wellness Institute (NWI) in 1977. The NWI has remained active, and continues to endorse the positive correlation between healthy, balanced lifestyle and wellness.

As the twentieth century waned, the rigid status quo of the medical field began to come under further pressure. Despite the undeniable impact of the biomedical model, there are those who feel that the disconnect between it and other causes and treatments is far too vast. In fact, there was a feeling that the biomedical model actually fell short when trying to explain illness. It was surmised that the problem "stems partly from three assumptions: all illness has a single underlying cause, disease (pathology) is always the single cause, and removal or attenuation of the disease will result in a return to health. Evidence exists that all three assumptions are wrong" (Do biomedical models, 2004). More specifically, psychiatrist George Engel expressed his lament with the tendency of medical field to discount anything other than biological issues when he noted that "classical science readily fostered the notion of the body as a machine, of disease as the consequence of breakdown of the machine, and of the doctor's task as repair of the machine" (Engel, 1977).

As a new century would dawn, it seemed that although the divide between traditional medicine and alternative treatment was still pretty wide, there could be some light at the end of the tunnel. Traditional practitioners were more apt to admit (even if grudgingly) that there was possibly a place for alternative treatments in the management of their patients. Many actually began to embrace the wellness philosophy, and most would agree that people should take an active interest in their own well being. Continued shifting of this paradigm will allow the established medical community to realize that a human is not a being of separate parts, but instead a synergistic entity whose parts undeniably interface with each other.

As we close this section, it is probably important at this point to make an observation. While we have outlined how the biomedical model may be rather strict and inflexible when it concerns causes and treatments, we should emphatically underscore the importance and effectiveness of the model on mankind. What had begun as a radical departure from accepted practice regarding diagnosis and healing gave rise to an ability to identify and remove a number of diseases ... many chronic diseases were eliminated, while others had been dramatically suppressed. I would submit that everyone reading this book has been a beneficiary of the traditional medicine tract, which we now know is not all that old in the course of history. What has been the impact of these advances on public health? The results have proven nothing short of dramatic. To illustrate, from 1900 to 2014, amazingly life expectancy in the United States had increased from 47 years to 79 years (Health, United States, 2015). Without a doubt, much of this impact can be attributed to the evolution of biomedicine.

Wellness 2000 CE - Present

As the wellness seesaw continues to swing back and forth entering the 21st century, new terminology and new approaches to wellness are becoming commonplace. In an effort to tag new approaches to health care, descriptive terms such as *complementary medicine* and *alternative medicine* have become common. In fact, they are often combined into the term *Complementary and Alternative Medicine,* or *CAM*. Although the terms *complementary* and *alternative* are often used to mean the same thing, they do actually represent two different ideas.

At the risk of playing a frustrating game of semantics with you, I will try to separate these terms. Alternative medicine is considered to have positive effects like medicine, but has not been verified by scientific studies. A method that is truly alternative is a non-traditional method used *instead* of traditional treatment, and is very rarely used. For instance, someone who has been diagnosed with cancer and decides to go to a cabin in the mountains and meditate all day in the fresh air, while taking no medicine or other treatments, could be considered to be using alternative methods.

Complimentary health care is using alternative medicine / alternative practices *along with* traditional medical practices, with the theory being that one will improve the other. The most common complimentary medicine includes supplements such as vitamins, minerals, and herbs. In addition, practices that focus on

165

various parts of the mind and body are considered complimentary, such as yoga, tai chi, massage, and chiropractic. If our cancer patient above decided to have a daily massage and acupuncture before going to the cabin to meditate, they would be involved in complimentary treatment.

Do people really use complementary and alternative methods and practices? It would seem so:

- A 2007 study by the NCCIH found that nearly 38 percent of adults in the US and 12 percent of children were employing some form of CAM (The Use of Complementary, 2008).
- A 2010 study conducted by the AARP/NCCAM found that 53 percent of people over 50 years old had used CAM methods during their lives, with 47 percent saying they had tried CAM in the previous 12 month period (Complementary and Alternative Medicine, 2011).
- In 2007, adults in the United States spent $33.9 billion out of pocket on visits to CAM practitioners and purchases of CAM products, classes, and materials ... 38.1 million adults made an estimated 354.2 million visits to practitioners of CAM (U.S. Department of Health, 2009).

If numbers such as these continue to trend, it would stand to reason that increasing numbers of people are employing non-traditional strategies to assist them in their search for personal wellness.

As we begin to close this section, I would be remiss if I didn't mention another term: *integrative medicine*. Integrative medicine seems to be a logical progression, since it marries *scientifically proven practices* from the fields of traditional medicine with those from complementary and alternative therapies to produce a comprehensive health plan. It is healing oriented, and deals with the total person (body, mind, and spirit). It also promotes healthy living, prevention of illness, and the creation of a partnership with medical professionals. It remains to be seen how integrative health care is embraced, but in my mind, integrative health care seems to best represent the truest spirit of wellness.

So there it is ... congratulations on surviving the trip across 5,000 years of wellness! Of particular interest to me is the ebb and flow of something resembling a *wellness concept* throughout history. It almost seems as though wellness has swung back and forth like the pendulum on a clock, fluctuating between traditional and non-traditional approaches. Currently, the CAM (Complimentary and Alternative Method) approach is in vogue, combining some elements of both in an attempt to achieve the elusive wellness balance. Yet, if history has shown us anything, change is constant, so it will be intriguing to see what the next pass of the pendulum reveals. Will it move toward the more comprehensive integrative health care? Only time will tell.

Regardless, with so much of life out of your control, you must remember that wellness is your chance to take responsibility for the quality of your life through the choices you make. Recall for a moment my favorite definition of wellness: *"an active process of becoming aware of, and making choices toward, a more successful existence."* You can and should become more aware of your health, and subsequently make the good choices to create a more successful existence for yourself.

Personally ...

Speaking of complementary and alternative practices ... recently I was called to serve on jury duty. Huh? (I know, but stick with me.) Like most of you, I can think of a lot of things I would rather be doing than jury duty ... but I showed up at the appointed time to fulfill my civic responsibility. I know it's important to go to jury duty... because at the courthouse they told me and 100 of my newest friends that it was important ... because if we didn't show up, the justice system won't work ... our constitution ... trial by peers ... if not for us being there, over 20 cases would not have resulted in pleas that very morning. Oh, by the way ... there's coffee over here ... coffee over there ... we'll make more coffee if you need more coffee ... there's a soda machine if you don't drink coffee ... if you like to smoke while you drink coffee, the smoking areas are out that door ... blah, blah, blah! It seems that the courthouse employees (who all appear to be frustrated, out of work stand-up comedians) must be paid a subsidy by the caffeine and nicotine industries to promote the unhealthiest lifestyles possible! Sheesh, I'm here, I'm a captive audience, let's move on! Hahaha ... but to my point ...

As usual, time stands still waiting for this judge or that judge to send down their docket. As luck would have it, my number was pulled for pre-trial interrogation by lawyers. The lawsuit dealt with a car accident and the damages incurred, and one of the questions asked of me and 14 other bright eyed prospective jurors was regarding chiropractors and chiropractic care. I found the responses intriguing. I was the only one who had positive experiences with chiropractic. Two others had gone to chiropractors, but noticed no difference; the other twelve had never gone to a chiropractor, but felt comfortable completely hammering the profession and its practitioners. If my new acquaintances are any indication, many complementary and alternative practices still have a long way to go to be accepted! Oh, and despite how important I was ... regardless of my vital importance to the entire process of jurisprudence in our republic ... at the risk of anarchy and civil disobedience ... I wasn't selected for the jury either! Hahaha ...

The Wellness Pie

We noted during our fifty century excursion above that for centuries, healing typically incorporated whole body tactics. As science became more refined, the approach shifted to a more body-centric plan. Based on everything we see now, there is a new acceptance (or re-acceptance) of non-traditional methods to augment health and wellness. It should also be clear that wellness is more than just a cholesterol level, a blood sugar reading, or the number on a bathroom scale. It also seems obvious that the term "wellness" represents a more holistic theory, meaning that it is characterized by the treatment of the entire person, taking into account social, mental, and spiritual factors as well as physical ones.

In an effort to grasp the overall concept of wellness more thoroughly, it often helps to visualize a pie that has been cut in equal slices. There are a number of wellness gurus that have a pie with eight slices, some with seven, some with ten ... I like six. My book ... my pie. The six slices each represent a different aspect of your being. In my pie, the slices can be labeled as *emotional, occupational, spiritual, intellectual, social,* and *physical.* You should strive to achieve balance both *within* and *between* all areas to maximize your wellness. Remember that baking a good pie depends on the interaction of all the ingredients to attain the finished product. The same is true of the wellness pie that is presented here. The balance between the various dimensions of your life will allow you to achieve the wellness you seek. I am certainly not a recognized expert on these areas, but as a means of increasing topical understanding, I can offer you a few pearls of wisdom regarding each piece of the pie. Off we go!

Emotional Wellness

"To me, good health is more than just exercise and diet. It's really a point of view and a mental attitude you have about yourself."
Albert Schweitzer (physician, missionary, Nobel prize winner)

I'm sure it's not a surprise to hear that everyone faces challenges. Let's face it, life can be tough, and not always what we consider fair. We are always being exposed to situations that cause anxiety, stress, and sadness. It would not shock the reader to know that every person handles stress differently, and also that everyone has a variety of success when it comes to juggling the responsibilities of life, family, friends, work, and the medley of other obligations we face.

A person's *emotional wellness* (sometimes referred to as "psychological" or "mental" wellness) can be considered as their ability to successfully negotiate the many struggles of life, while simultaneously maintaining a positive outlook. In other words, emotional wellness is a measure of how adept we are at having an awareness and acceptance of our own inner feelings, as well as an understanding that life is sometimes frustrating … all the while maintaining the ability to be an optimist about the whole mess.

With this in mind, why is it that we will immediately react to a physical ailment, but tend to downplay (or even hide) an emotional issue? For example, we will toss down aspirin for sore muscles or a headache, or wrap a sore joint with an elastic brace. If that doesn't work, it's off to the physician for help. Yet, many of us will have problems discerning issues with our feelings ... even if we inherently know that something is out of kilter in that area, we either don't know what to do about it ourselves or are very hesitant to find help from professionals. Recalling that overall wellness is achieved by a balance of all areas, it is mandatory we recognize that our emotional health encroaches on our overall wellness *at least* as much as our physical condition does.

Similar to the dichotomy between health and wellness, it must also be observed that the state of *not* having psychological issues such as stress, anxiety or depression does not necessarily indicate emotional wellness. Even though we all know that you can't possibly feel good all of the time, we still strive to do things that make us feel good. Along with the two constants death and taxes, it is also guaranteed that you will encounter a loss or some hurt feelings along the way. It is your effectiveness in being able to manage these situations that keeps you balanced ... in psychological terms that capability is known as *resilience*.

Resilience is defined as "that ineffable quality that allows some people to be knocked down by life and come back stronger than ever" (Psychology Today). I prefer to think of those with resilience as those who can "improvise, adapt, and overcome." While that phrase certainly is an unofficial mantra of the United States Marine Corps, it also represents what needs to happen for you to achieve and maintain emotional wellness. To me, this "well" contingent seems self confident, and flexible enough to learn and listen to other views than their own. The inevitable brush with stress does not disable them, but rather they face it head on and make the best of whatever gets tossed at them. They are generally content, and are often defined by their ability to laugh and have fun. In short, they can best be described as exhibiting what the French term as *joie de vivre,* or the *joy of living.*

Since the target audience of this book is the obese cohort, this is a good time to mention body image as it relates to emotional health. There is no doubt that we live in a very visual culture. As such, there are certain norms that people are supposed to conform to. I affectionately refer to this as the *Barbie Paradigm* and the *G.I. Joe Paradigm.* Much like the favorite girls play toy, *Barbie women* should have impossibly proportionate hips / chest to waist ratios. Men don't get a break here either, since they are expected to be extremely muscular with almost no body fat, just like the action figure that they grew up with. These unrealistic beliefs exacerbate body image issues exponentially with the obese.

Speaking more in macro terms, the perceived fat fight has created a number of obsessed, compulsive people ... many of whom are emotional wrecks. These people face discrimination, and often suffer with eating disorders. They constantly worry about getting ... or being ... fat. All the while, the supposed reward for this is the achievement of the perfect proportion. There are countless studies that show being thin does not necessarily equate to a happiness level. As we know (or are at least hopefully learning from this book), wellness is achieved through a balance of many facets, with body image only being a small portion. Let's be honest, bodies are as unique as snowflakes. When you recognize that your body is yours and yours alone, it aids in positive self image. Although one of the prime reasons I wrote this book was to relay an effective way to gain control of your eating for life, wellness can be achieved regardless of size.

Knowing that, one of the absolute best ways to maintain healthy emotional wellness is to ... TAKE CARE OF YOUR BODY! That's right, your body's health affects your emotional health ... which in turn affects the body's health ... which will affect your emotional health ... okay, you get the picture. I just wanted to reinforce the symbiotic relationship between all facets of the body yet again. Although we discuss the effects of workouts in further depth in other sections of this book, suffice to know that purely from a physiological point of view, working out causes the body to release *endorphins*. As you probably know, endorphins are actually "*endogenous opioid neuropeptides*" ... ummm, okay, let's forget that. Maybe we could say that endorphins function to transmit the electrical signals in your brain. Not feeling that either? How's this ... they operate like opiate type drugs (morphine, codeine, etc.) in that they mask pain and stress naturally, only without the addiction of opiates? Okay, as simple as we can put it ... the stuff the body releases in a workout makes you feel good! Of course, other byproducts of working out include shaping the body as you want it, fitting in your clothes, liking the reflection in the mirror a little more, etc. ... all of which contribute to feeling better. So in concluding the section on emotional wellness, we again see the critical interdependency of each piece of our wellness pie. From an emotional wellness perspective (and with all due apologies to the 1967 movie classic *Cool Hand Luke*), it is the acquisition of balance that allows you to "get your mind right!"

Personally...

Emotionally, I firmly believe that one of the biggest assets that a person can possess is the ability to laugh ... particularly at themselves. Too many people worry too much, especially about things they can't control. Lighten up a little bit. Here is a fact ... you aren't all that important ... like the rest of us, you are quickly replaceable. Don't take yourself so seriously.

Occupational Wellness

"Never continue in a job you don't enjoy. If you're happy in what you're doing, you'll like yourself, you'll have inner peace. And if you have that, along with physical health, you will have had more success than you could possibly have imagined."
Johnny Carson (television host, comedian)

What Is Occupational Wellness?

There is no doubt that the majority of us are intimately familiar with work. We either work now ... have worked ... are looking for work ... work part time ... are working but really want to do some other kind of work ... or any number of other combinations regarding ... work. Let's face it, we may not be completely enamored with it, but we generally understand that work is at the very least a "necessary evil." With that in mind, here's a sobering statistic ... working consumes roughly one quarter of the average person's week. That doesn't include overtime, or traveling to work, or preparing for work, or thinking about work ... that is just *being* at work! Ugh. Since sleep takes up about another quarter of your week, half of your week is gone before you even consider doing anything for fun! Consequently, it should be obvious that your choice of occupation can (and does) have a dramatic effect on your overall wellness. As such, it behooves us to constantly strive to achieve a certain level of *occupational wellness*.

Loosely defined, occupational wellness is considered *how the work that we do makes us feel*. Of course, there is more to it than

179

that. Occupational wellness takes into account your ability to handle the daily rigors of your job, how well you can balance your work and leisure time, and also whether you achieve some satisfaction both personally and financially through your job. All of these things contribute to your occupational wellness, your balance, and ... your slice of pie!

You and Your Occupation

Today's workers face a different set of stressors than workers in the past. In the "old days", the average middle class person tried to get a job with the government or some big company, stay there thirty years, retire with a gold watch and draw a check monthly for the rest of their lives. More often than not, you chose a job or career path because of opportunity, not necessarily because it was your dream. For instance, Uncle Sal had worked at "the plant" for 26 years and could get you on. So whether you liked the work or not, you clocked in and clocked out, never really considering your job related wellness. While this option still exists, it is <u>much</u> less prevalent than in the past.

Without getting too socio-economic about it, this paradigm has changed for a number of reasons. First, many of the "thirty year" jobs … such as those in the steel, automobile, and textile industries … have left this country and may never return. Also, much like people moving from farms to factories in the Industrial Revolution, the explosion of technology has reduced the need for many traditional "blue collar" workers. As the employment landscape changed, employees found that without access to as many jobs with longevity, benefits, and retirement plans, their future was not so bright. One result of this realization was the creation of portable personal retirement accounts (i.e. 401k plans) which allows the worker to contribute to their own retirement regardless of where they work. The loyal "company man" of days gone by has been replaced by employees who leverage pay scales, benefits, and working conditions. While things such as job security and employment longevity used to rank as top considerations, they are far down the wish list for many current job seekers. For instance, in 2012 the average length of stay at a job was 4.6 years (Employee Tenure Summary, 2014) ... among those workers born from 1977-1997 (the "Millennials"), their expectations for a job is to only be there for less than three years.

Okay, we can agree that it's likely you will have quite a few jobs in your career. Armed with this knowledge, it becomes pretty apparent that the best way to achieve occupational wellness is to find a job (or jobs) that will provide satisfaction and gratification. During the job search, be honest with yourself. Examine your talents and skills, as well as any other requirements you may have (certain shifts, days of the week, pay scale, etc.). When you have a fair idea of what you would find interesting and rewarding, it may be easier to find a job that proves satisfying. At the very least it should narrow your search considerably. You should seek something that you want to do, that allows room for progress, and is interesting and motivating. It should also allow you enough time off to enjoy outside hobbies, and give you the feeling that you are an important part of accomplishing something.

Matching your talents, skills, and desires to the right occupation can be a daunting task ... it could even be considered a real pain in the rear. After you find a suitable job opportunity, go wow the prospective employer with your interview brilliance, and you will undoubtedly get the job. Now what? Well, most bosses find that if someone has a good work ethic and integrity, they already have a lot of the problems behind them. So work hard, be honest, and do what is asked. Sounds like common sense, but as the saying goes "Common sense ain't so common anymore." Also, communicate effectively, since a large percentage of problems occur from communication breakdowns. In addition, there is a marked difference in hearing and listening ... everybody hears, but not everyone listens. Work on that skill. This is a great start at keeping the boss happy.

What about your on-the-job wellness? Following the "glass half full" theory, be positive and look for benefits in your job. Your place of employment owes you a safe workplace, and if you've done your homework, you'll know whether the pay they offer is satisfactory. Beyond that, you should strive to be a problem solver, whether as a member of a team or by going solo. If you identify a problem, don't just complain, have several solutions available. It is imperative that you increase your skill sets related to your position, so look for training and learning opportunities. Remembering the great wellness information you've read here (a shameless plug for the book by the way), try to maintain a healthy equilibrium between your occupation and the rest of your life ... remember that increased balance increases wellness. The old adage *"All work and no play makes Jack a dull boy"* is more than just a saying ... too much work is not in keeping with a healthy lifestyle balance. Above all, don't feel the need to just "settle" in your job. If it isn't what you envisioned, remain motivated, take small steps, and keep striving for your goal. Give yourself a chance for success. It is awfully hard to find the perfect job that you feel is enjoyable to attend and is financially and intrinsically rewarding ... however, the saddest part is if you stop *trying* to find it. Life is too short to be miserable at work.

As everyone knows, one of the most important things about a job is the salary ... how much does it pay? No doubt pay is important, but the pay itself is in no way a guarantee of occupational wellness. I can hear it now ... "Okay Bruce, pay doesn't matter ... that's just plain stupid!" I'll pause here while you laugh ... and curse ... and throw the book. Now that you feel better, I want to tell you that many people choose jobs that pay little or nothing, and many actually get tremendous satisfaction from volunteer positions. To illustrate my point about jobs and pay, I give you ... the President of the United States! The most powerful person in the world currently makes $400,000 a year. I know that's not peanuts ... and yes, I know that everything from housing to haircuts is paid for by the taxpayer ... and I realize there are about a zillion other perks that go with the job. But for the stress of a 24 hour a day, 7 day a week job the pay seems pretty paltry. If it's not money, what drives someone to seek the top job? Things like ego, power, legacy ...who knows what the whole list is. The one thing I do know ... the leader of the free world ... the person who could end life as we know it with a few phone calls and button pushes ... works for a salary that is about $45 an hour. You'll never convince me it's about the money!

Regardless of your job choice ... whether it is just a temporary stop along the way or the perfect career choice ... you should always, always, always do the best that you can. Of course, this is important to kiss the boss's butt, but it is even more important for your self-satisfaction. If you leave work at the end of the day knowing you did your best, you will have earned both money and intrinsic reward. Dr. Martin Luther King Jr. summarized this idea best when he said *"If a man is called to be a street sweeper, he should sweep streets even as a Michelangelo painted, or Beethoven composed music, or Shakespeare wrote poetry. He should sweep streets so well that all the hosts of heaven and earth will pause to say, 'Here lived a great street sweeper who did his job well."* Now THAT would be the epitome of occupational wellness!

Personally ...

Frankly, I can quiz almost everyone I know regarding their theory on occupational wellness, and their answers all distill down to one over-riding statement. Simply put ... _"If they quit payin', I quit goin'."_ Self explanatory ... work is like a colonoscopy ... not always pleasant but something most all of us have to endure in an effort to make life better. I never was particularly enchanted with any job I ever had, other than to understand that it was a means to an end. Generally speaking, I also never hated to go to work either. Maybe that was a sign that I had achieved a certain amount of wellness (in an occupational sense).

Spiritual Wellness

"Just as a candle cannot burn without fire, men cannot live without a spiritual life." Buddha

Picture this ... one night, sometime in the dark, distant past, our ancestors were just hanging out around the cave. Our great grandfathers (many times over) relaxed with bellies full of freshly killed, cooked, and eaten prehistoric beast. Their women had swept the cave, thrown the bones onto the fire, and put the young to sleep. The fire had been stoked for the night to keep the cave warm and to chase critters away, so now our distant kinfolk could wrap up in some stinky animal skins for the night. As they looked up at the twinkling lights in the sky above them, for at least a brief moment, they undoubtedly wondered why they were there, and questioned what their purpose was. In essence, they were trying to understand the dimension we refer to as spirituality.

Naturally, it would have been tough to ponder hazy topics such as spirituality when you spent your entire day and night trying to avoid becoming a meal yourself. As people gradually acquired enough food, shelter, and security to allow themselves a few moments to think about the grand scheme of things, they certainly would have wondered how they fit into the world around them. This ability to reason has always been what humans have done ... they have the unique cognitive ability to reflect on themselves. In fact, this ability for abstract thought separates us from animals ... well, that and the opposable thumb thing!

To me, there is no doubt that of all the slabs of my wellness pie, the most difficult of all the six dimensions to define and develop is spiritual wellness. You want bigger biceps, you perform exercises that pull weight toward the body. A healthier spirit? Ummm ... not as easy to answer. Yet, regardless of these problems, you cannot discount the value of spiritual wellness, since it is a major contributor to the overall wellness that we should all seek. It's kind of ironic that many thousand years later, we are still searching for meaning and purpose exactly like our forebears did (well, except for the cave ... and the fire ... and the bones ... and the stinky furs).

What is Spiritual Wellness?

It would seem that our first task is to try to explain this spiritual wellness stuff. That is very, very, very easy to do, since spirituality is ... different for everyone! Soooo ... let's try to agree on a few points. First, we will assume that spiritual wellness is the ultimate goal that results from your attempt to develop spiritually. I suppose we can say that spiritual wellness could loosely be considered the *process of searching for a meaning to our existence.* So far, so good. Across the continuum of human existence, this quest for meaning has resulted in endless theories, and has been addressed by countless experts in fields like theology, science, and philosophy. All those folks are much smarter than I'll ever be, so if you feel moved to do research, have at it ... you'll find more information than you could ever hope to read. As for me, I'll just try to give the reader a basic interpretation of this stuff.

Let's take a crack at it ... maybe we can think of spiritual wellness as ... a sort of recipe! How's that for a stretch? Start with one part of the *ability to ask major questions about life's purpose,* then add a generous amount of *concern for a universal system of values,* and mix it together with a *sense of what is right and wrong.* Blend into this mixture a *dash of caring about the welfare of others,* and then stir in equal parts *compassion, forgiveness, and tolerance.* Finally, sprinkle in a dose of *acceptance for the things that occur that cannot be understood in absolute terms.* Sift this all together with the *intention*

189

to improve the world, as well as to improve yourself. Allow the product to simmer throughout your lifetime, seasoning along the way with your own *morals, ethics, principles, standards, mores, and values.* Voila...spiritual wellness!

Of course, your recipe might yield something that looks totally different than mine ... since everyone is different, their spiritual wellness will manifest itself differently too. Important to know is that your spiritual wellness comes from within you, so resist the temptation to compare / contrast what you need for your balance with what others may need. Also, remember that whatever gives you wellness in a spiritual sense, you must strive to achieve it for your maximum overall balance.

Spiritual or Religious

It would be impossible to discuss spiritual well being without mentioning differences between religion and spirituality. It must be noted that being well spiritually does not necessarily mean being religious ... although religion is spiritual and spirituality is religious. Huh? I know, very vague, and we're only scratching the surface.

Although some folks use the terms religion and spirituality interchangeably, most people have at least some concept that there are differences between the two. *Religion* is generally thought of as a set of beliefs, views, and practices shared by a social group, community, or culture. It was created by human beings, and requires members to follow a particular doctrine, as well as to participate in formal practices. *Spirituality* is normally practiced individually, can be manifested in any number of forms, and follows no particular formalities. Typically, spirituality stresses peace, compassion, and the meaning of life, while recognizing the existence of a greater power. Maybe this will help ... an easy but simple to understand comparison ... according to one website (What is spirituality? 2015), the relationship between spirituality and religion resembles a game of Aussie football (or soccer as it's known in the U.S.). In this comparison, religion is characterized as a formal game of soccer, with teams, rules, referees, a marked field, etc. On the other hand, spirituality can be considered as a person kicking a soccer ball around, not necessarily on any field or with any official rules, but still getting the essence of the game. Simple analogy, but spot on.

Armed with some basic descriptions, we can now go a little further. For instance, we can ask if spirituality by itself would be enough ... can it stand alone? Rabbi David Wolpe (Wolpe, 2013) feels that the religion serves a greater purpose as he notes "institutions are also the only mechanism human beings know to perpetuate ideologies and actions. If books were enough, why have universities? If guns enough, why have a military? If self-governance enough, let's get rid of Washington." He goes on to say that "people's internal sense of goodness does not always match their behavior" and also that "Being religious does not mean you have to agree with all the positions and practices of your own group." The good rabbi gives a compelling argument for the importance of religion, feeling that its structure and accountability help to keep people on track.

Comparatively, there are arguments equally as compelling for the theory of spiritualism. For instance, the 14th Dalai Lama, leader of Tibetan Buddhism, feels that the individual should strive to be spiritual because "spirituality is concerned with those qualities of the human spirit – such as love and compassion, patience, tolerance, forgiveness, contentment, a sense of responsibility, a sense of harmony – which brings happiness to both self and others." Consequently he feels that religion is more ideological, and doesn't necessarily guarantee happiness, which is

192

apparent as he notes that "This is why I sometimes say religion is something we can perhaps do without. What we cannot do without are these basic spiritual qualities" (Stephenson, 2016). Another viewpoint comes from doctor and philosopher Deepak Chopra, who sums up his view of the difference in religion and spirituality by saying that "Religion is belief in someone else's experience. Spirituality is having your own experience" (Khan, 2015).

While you try to wrap your head around the two concepts, let me toss a third group in the mix. There is a group who considers themselves *Spiritual But Not Religious* (or *SBNR*). This group is worth mentioning, primarily because it is growing, and growing fairly quickly. In fact, a Pew Research poll ("Nones" on the Rise, 2012) found that one fifth of the United States public is not affiliated with any religion … even more dramatic is the fact that a full *one third* of those under thirty years old also do not claim any affiliation. Of the unattached group, thirty seven percent claim to be SBNR … that's right, spiritual but not religious. SBNRs may actually be the logical evolution of the estimated 30% of baby boomers (Steinfels, 1993) who identify as *believers, not belongers*, claiming to remain very inquisitive about religion, yet avoiding religious groups. Regardless of terminology, they form a portion of society that tries to meld parts of both the spiritual and the religious into some form of philosophical ideal.

Regardless of the causes, just a friendly word of advice for all those who are locked in to the "my way or the highway" paradigm. Whether you choose to follow religion, spirituality, SBNR, or somewhere else along the imaginary line, instead of demonizing others, exhibit a healthy dose of tolerance. Please respect everyone's freedom to follow or ignore any path they may choose. More importantly, understand that it is difficult to take someone seriously when they say they cannot tolerate a view other than theirs because the other view is so ... INTOLERANT! Pot, meet the kettle. After all, regardless of your beliefs, tolerance is a very noble universal concept!

Religion or spirituality ... spirituality or religion ... I've tossed it out there for your consideration. Which path suits you? Certainly, the disparity between the two is not set in stone. Just maybe ... could it be that neither religion nor spirituality could exist without the other? Father James Martin (2012) thinks so, stating that "being spiritual and being religious are *both* part of being in relationship with God." He continues, "Religion without spirituality becomes a dry list of dogmatic statements divorced from the life of the spirit", and also adds that "spirituality without religion can become a self-centered complacency divorced from the wisdom of a community." Makes a lot of sense.

So now, I hope you're ready, because here comes my next brilliant observation! The words *religion* and *spirituality* are just that ... words. I certainly am not one to threaten, cajole, browbeat, domineer, intimidate, menace, entice, flatter, induce, or persuade when it comes to your spiritual wellness. As you know by now, my main concern is for your spiritual wellness as it relates to the complete wellness pie. Spiritual wellness needs to be nurtured for your overall balance. The path you choose to travel to achieve this balance is largely up to you. However, it seems that instead of getting so caught up in the terms, we should remember that good people aren't good because of words, but rather in how they walk through life. To close and sum up, Linda Mercadante (2014) notes that we are all *"in danger of becoming rigid or comatose, inflexible or numb. All of us need to find ways to develop and live our faith in the company of others."* Hmmm ... we need to find ways to live our faith in the company of others? I think we may be on to something.

Spiritual Wellness and Your Health

Following the general path we've established, balanced life often leads to some increased level of wellness. So then, being "well" in a spiritual sense should result in the ownership of inner peace, which serves as an added buffer to life's bumps. Having said that, does spiritual wellness actually have any cross-over effects that are beneficial to our physical well being too?

With apologies to all my engineering friends (you know who you are), I detest books and papers that contain large amount of statistics ... boring! Having apologized, I must now admit that in this section, I caved in to the "dark side of the force" and have included statistics and numbers to support that a correlation exists regarding health and spiritual wellness. The following chunks of information are fairly painless to read ... while perusing these research conclusions, please take a second to absorb the impact of each:

- Reports show that between 60% - 90% of all visits to healthcare professionals result from stress related issues. Since it is accepted that religion / spirituality reduces stress, it seems obvious that a cause / effect relationship exists (Puchalski, 2001).

- A heart transplant study showed that patients who took part in religious activities complied better with follow-up treatment, had improved physical functioning at the 12-month follow-up visit, had higher levels of self-esteem, and had less anxiety and fewer health worries (Puchalski, 2001).

- After an examination of over 300 studies on the relationship between health and spirituality, close to 80 percent of the studies "find significantly higher well-being among those who are more spiritual" (Rasmus, 2013).

- A questionnaire of hospitalized patients showed that the most commonly used non-drug method of controlling pain was prayer. With 76% of the patients reporting the use of prayer to help them cope, it was used more often than intravenous pain medication (66%), pain injections (62%), relaxation (33%), touch (19%), and massage (9%) (Puchalski, 2001).

- "Religiosity" seems to be a predictor of survival, with the frequent religious service attendees averaging a 37% higher survival rate. It is interesting to note that this increase is equal to the affects of cholesterol lowering drugs or cardio rehabilitation exercise (Koenig, 2012).

- Much research operates on the assumption that if spirituality is beneficial to health, mortality rates should reflect it. Associated studies find that there is indeed a correlation, showing that 68% found increased religious / spirituality involvement equaled greater longevity (Koenig, 2012).

- Weekly religious service attendance correlated to a 46% mortality reduction. Even controlling for a variety of factors (age, race, sickness level, and other health and social factors) mortality was still reduced by 28%. (Spirituality May Help)

197

- Religious beliefs and associated activities "are associated with more positive psychological outcomes, because these beliefs and activities give meaning to life events, especially difficult ones" and that "In the big picture, spirituality is the greatest source of thriving, resilience and flourishing in the human condition" (Rasmus, 2013).

- Some observational studies suggest that people who have regular spiritual practices tend to live longer. The bulk of statistical evidence seems to validate the theory that those practicing religion follow better health practices, and there are a number of possibilities as to why. Some plausible reasons include: peer influence, increased self-esteem, increased sense of perceived control, prescribed practices, and a general philosophical outlook that values social ties and treating one's body with respect (Strawbridge, et al, 1997)

Alright, I'll stop. Hopefully you slogged through these facts and stats. Based on the research noted here (along with much more), several things become apparent. First, it seems that integrating spirituality into patient health care increases the quality of the care. Also, since balance in life is a goal to achieve wellness, then it would logically follow that those who have addressed their spiritual wellness have already taken a big step toward overall wellness.

Well, it is time to tie up this section on spiritual wellness. As I warned you earlier, the concepts regarding spiritual wellness are sometimes obscure and murky. We have outlined that *spiritual* is not necessarily the same as *religious*, but that the two concepts often lead to the same result. The outright importance of spiritual wellness is noteworthy because it contributes to your total wellness. Even more, spiritual wellness is a dynamic experience that can help you find meaning and purpose in your life. Your interface with your spiritual being may come from prayer, meditation, practices, or a hundred other ways. As for me, I prefer attending church and following the associated practices, since it all serves a purpose similar to rebooting my computer ... I feel "reset" and ready to face life's challenges. My inner spiritual wellness meter also tells me that the world would be far better off if we all would only follow the *Golden Rule* and *Ten Commandments*, regardless of religious beliefs, affiliations, or spirituality level. Regardless, in my experience, most people really do want to know the meaning of life. So I will apologize for sounding like some guy dressed in a toga sitting on top of a snow covered mountain in Tibet, but exploring and expanding your spiritual wellness can go a long way toward answering the questions of life for you.

If you are so inclined, on a clear night, step outside and look up at the countless twinkling lights in the sky. If you concentrate on the shimmering beacons above, you may even feel the same sense of wonder and awe that our ancestors in the cave did. You too might even be moved to pause for a second and open your mind to ponder your place in the universe. If you're really, really in tune to your senses, you may even be able to smell the distant aroma of the meat cooking on your ancestor's fire thousands of years ago ... of course, that could just be the next door neighbor grilling!

Personally...

As I mentioned elsewhere in this book, I was born in the south, and have lived there my entire life. Religion was important, and Protestant churches were everywhere. In fact, if you take away the churches, banks, hair salons, and auto parts stores, I firmly believe many southern towns would fold up! It was somewhere around my senior year in high school that my "religious slump" began, and I decided not to attend church. As an excuse, I used the fact that the same people I see drinking and dancing on Saturday night were the ones in the front row of the church on Sunday. I justified that they were hypocrites, and as a result, I wouldn't have anything to do with a church that allowed that! Of course, as time passed, life happened to me as it does to everyone. Along the way I began to ask those higher order questions about purpose, reason, etc. During this period, I realized that the problem was not with the church I had attended ... or with the religious path and doctrine that the church followed ... or even with those heathen drinking dancers sitting in the front row! No, the problem was inside me. I came to realize that those front row villains were indeed flawed ... with that knowledge, I also realized that they were in the perfect place on Sunday morning ... they were in the church. They were giving spiritual wellness their best shot by going to a place of religion, looking for guidance and support from the religious community. It is certainly not my place to pass judgment on those folks, since I have a full time job trying to keep myself in a state of spiritual wellness! After all, who needs to be in church more than people who have flaws?

Intellectual Wellness

"Man's mind, once stretched by a new idea,
never regains its original dimensions."
Oliver Wendell Holmes (lawyer, judge, Supreme Court Justice)

The term "intellect" loosely refers to a person's mental powers; more directly, their ability to understand, think, and reason, as well as their capacity for knowledge. Naturally it follows that *intellectual wellness* is the relative strength of an individual's mental capacity. Dr. Bill Hettler sums it up by stating that "intellectual wellness is stimulating the mind for stimulation sake" (Hettler, 1984). From my viewpoint, the concept of intellectual wellness is actually simple … intellectual wellness encourages you to learn.

Certainly, any conversation that includes terms like "mental capacity" must undoubtedly begin with a discussion of the brain. While there is still so much about the human brain that is unknown, we do know the brain controls bodily functions, as well as our intellectual being. While it is a sophisticated and complex organ, it needs exercise like all of our other organs to maintain its health … our brains will atrophy without exercise just as surely as our muscles do. Although the average person experiences a decline in the number of brain cells as they age (beginning somewhere in their mid twenties), scientists assure us that we will make neurons the rest of our lives … most importantly, this may happen in proportion to how much and how often we challenge our brains. Since neurons serve to connect with other cells and transmit info between, our intellectual wellness is directly affected by their function. By regularly stimulating the brain, we can continue to strengthen the neural connectors and retain our mental acuity.

Armed with the knowledge that we can affect our mental condition, wouldn't it be great to build some sort of mental backup that your body could rely on to help you withstand the effects of aging? The good news is that there has been substantial research showing that a variety of factors (including education levels, occupation, social interaction, etc.) may help to aid the creation of a certain kind of mental stockpile. It seems scientists believe that mental stimulation results in the formation of a "cognitive reserve" that helps you retain your mental abilities as you age. They surmise that this cognitive reserve concept helps to illustrate why some people are better able to cope with and tolerate changes in the brain as they age. In essence, your brain gets better at battling neurological damage due to aging and other factors, while at the same time showing little evidence of slowing down or memory loss. On a more micro level, much research has concluded that cognitive reserve can actually be divided into two portions: *brain reserve* and *cognitive reserve*. Though not meant to supply a comprehensive study of brain function, I'll tell you the difference as I understand it.

Brain reserve can be considered anatomical, and considers

brain size, the density of neurons and synapses that connect everything up there ... you know, brain stuff. Brain reserve also considers the proficiency of the brain to manage advancing damage, yet still function satisfactorily. On the flip side, cognitive reserve can be thought of as theoretical, looking at the possibility of making the pathways that are already there more efficient through various training methods ... it wants to focus on how the brain uses its resources when they are impaired. Further study and understanding of a cognitive reserve may help create methods to reduce the various dementia related problems experienced by so many.

How Can I Improve My Intellectual Wellness?

What can the average person do to create a lifestyle that supports brain health? The options are endless. No single activity has been shown superior in enhancing your intellectual wellness ... almost anything considered "intellectual" can help to strengthen our minds. While learning has traditionally been thought of as being accomplished academically, there really are no rules. Wellness depends on a personal heap of both formal education and experiences gained through your life. In other words, it doesn't have to be just book learnin'! Wellness can also be fostered through hobbies, cultural involvement, and community interaction. Read anything ... anywhere ... anytime. Crossword puzzles and word games are great ... they force the brain to be active. Even something as simple as using your non-dominant hand causes the brain to concentrate and relearn movements ... do things like brushing your teeth with the OTHER hand! When driving to work or the store, take a different route. Be open-minded, and expose yourself to beliefs, cultures, knowledge, and ideas that are different than yours. Listening to music is also helpful, since it causes the brain to make sense of the patterns that it is being exposed to. Creativity and curiosity are your friends ... challenge your mind. The important thing is that you make a commitment, and recognize that learning is a life-long process.

While we have discussed the importance of mental activity

206

for brain stimulation and health, the impact of physical exercise on your intellect cannot be dismissed. In a perfect example of the interactive nature of our pie pieces, exercise provides possibly the best investment of your time when considering your cognitive health. Studies indicate that active people enhance their cognitive function, improving memory and attention span along the way. It is painfully obvious that a symbiotic relationship exists between mental and physical health ... in fact, exercise seems to reverse the effects of aging on the brain (Carr, 2014).

I know how you are ... now you want specifics ... what can we do physically to increase our mental acuity? The answer is to do what you would do to "train" the rest of your body. The best news is that to retain your mental acumen, you don't need to run a marathon. For a quick boost, do some form of aerobic activity for twenty minutes or so ... at least enough to raise your heart rate to 60 - 70 percent of your maximum heart rate. If you recall, there was more on heart rate in the Workout section (Chapter 6). You could accomplish this by using exercise machines, such as exercise bikes, treadmills, elliptical machines, etc. It could be through a resistance workout, performed quickly in a circuit fashion. Or it could be as simple as walking around the block. Research shows a workout can immediately boost your brain skills, and the reason is apparent ... if you get the heart pumping, your brain receives more blood flow and oxygen, which enriches the brain. Regardless of the type of workout, researchers generally agree that the cognitive benefits last for at least an hour after exercise. For increased health benefits, it is recommended that you do thirty minutes of physical activity per day, but even less proves beneficial.

When It Comes to Your Brain, Use Your Head

I know that many of you have heard it, and lots of you have probably even repeated it. For many years there has been an urban myth going around that people only use about ten percent of their brain capacity. While this fact is often tossed around, research has proven this statement as clearly false. I am certain that lots of folks out there hope that their mental ... umm, shortcomings ... are caused by some evolutionary misfire that made their brain able to only handle ten percent of its capability. I'm here to report that their limits are most likely for other reasons! Most researchers feel that while you might only use varying percentages of brain capacity at any one time, over a 24 hour period you would likely use 100 percent of your brain at some point. More likely, as Boyd (2008) suggests, "it's not that we use 10 percent of our brains, merely that we only understand about 10 percent of how it functions."

Although we make fun of this popular myth here, other surveys show that it is obvious people really don't know much about their brains. As much as people understand about what exercises are good, what blood pressure numbers are optimal, and where their good and bad cholesterol levels should be, they are equally as clueless when discussing the brain. For instance, one poll notes that U.S. residents think that only 36% of the population will develop brain disease during their life. In a sobering reality, 60% will actually develop some form of brain impairment (New survey finds Americans, 2011). Yet another survey finds that a full 71% of folks assume that brain disease strikes both sexes equally. This is not entirely true, since although both sexes are stricken, women are more likely to suffer from multiple sclerosis (Multiple sclerosis, 2015), while 50 percent more men are affected with Parkinson's disease (Parkinson's Disease, 2016). It is also common for most folks (74%) to assume that since Grandma or good old Uncle Bob was a little "wacky" when they got older, then mental skills automatically fade as we age. However, some skills (notably vocabulary and social wisdom) can actually increase with age (Helmuth, 2011).

A number of risks *have* been identified, including lifestyle issues such as improper diet, tobacco use, alcohol abuse, inadequate sleep, and a variety of emotional problems. Physically, conditions such as high blood pressure, low or high blood sugar, and high cholesterol can all have a marked effect on brain function. These conditions and their effects can all be controlled, reduced, or eliminated. This proves once again that you should have a relationship with your medical professional, since they can diagnose and treat your problems. So, it comes full circle again ... to maintain your intellectual function (and wellness), you must maintain optimum health, remain physically active, and challenge yourself mentally. If you do this, you will have done the best you can to influence the variables under your control.

While there is much still to be learned about our brains, whether our intelligence increases, is maintained, or declines with age has been studied for over a century. Regardless of the affects of adulthood on mental capacity, it is a fact that brains will change, just like all other components of the body. While cognitive decline is common, impairment is not obligatory. Remember that to maintain intellectual health, people should be curious ... should seek intellectual challenge and stimulation; should relish the prospect of mental growth ... should challenge their minds at every turn. If you recall that intellectual wellness is a subset of overall wellness and comprises one-sixth of the wellness pie, you will understand that each portion relies on the other for optimum effectiveness. Strive for balance intellectually, as well as within all the wellness facets. One thing that is abundantly clear ... nowhere is the statement "use it or lose it" more valid than when discussing our brains.

Personally ...

For me, intellectual wellness is achieved (or augmented) through embracing lifelong learning. That can be as simple as learning how to change a tail light in your old Chevy, taking a computer class, reading, doing crossword puzzles, playing mah jongg on the computer, etc. Heck, even writing a book is intellectual ... and the fact that you are reading this one is good for you too! I also spend a lot of time doing genealogy research, which I find sparks interest in my connection with the past and serves as an intellectual stimulant. Oh, and it also reminds me that as I age, I am hurtling toward becoming an "ancestor" myself! Just know that the human brain must be constantly exercised to maintain its wellness. We're all aging every day, but that is no reason to surrender. To quote Welsh poet Dylan Thomas, "*Do not go gentle into that good night, old age should burn and rave at close of day; rage, rage against the dying of the light.*"

Social Wellness

*"I fear the day that technology will surpass our human interaction.
The world will have a generation of idiots."*
Albert Einstein

Origins of Social Wellness

It is very possible that you have not heard of ... or at least
not thought much about ... the social wellness portion of the
wellness spectrum. In relation to the other components that we
discuss here, it is the newest ... yet certainly no less important
than the others. Honestly, I think that as a people, we are just
beginning to understand the importance of social wellness. While
there are endless definitions of the term social wellness, I kind of
like to think that it is simply *the ability to positively interact with
those around you.* Those who exhibit social health will give and
receive support from others, use good communication skills,
participate in their community, and respect themselves and
others. Although this may sound like some sort of condensed
version of a Boy Scout oath, it is well established that social
wellness has a profound effect on your health, both physically and
mentally.

To discuss social wellness, we first need to go back. Where
did this dependence on others begin? Remember our cave
dwelling ancestors that we discussed earlier? If you recall, when
we last visited, they were hanging out around the cave eating
meat, gazing at stars, and wondering what the heck they were

doing there! These folks certainly hadn't heard the term social wellness ... yet they understood that there was increased safety from animals and other humans with bad intentions because they were in a group. Just the fact that they were munching on some ribs would most likely indicate their reliance on social wellness ... I can assure you that getting this meat wasn't as easy as stopping by the local grocery store. It was a labor intensive, hands on process that would not have been possible without a high degree of social interaction.

Okay, so humans were pack animals in prehistory ... how does that impact us now? Mainly, the rudimentary social structure they created back then has continued to be refined throughout the following centuries, and the need for people to depend on others became normal. In fact, this new normal would become ingrained deeply in our instincts. The ancestors had correctly discovered that survival took food, water, and shelter. In addition, they also had figured out that without the interaction of others, their future chances were bleak. So, although we have climbed and clawed our way to the top of the evolutionary ladder, in some ways we are just like other creatures who still roam in packs, herds, gaggles, pods, flocks, prides, teams, and swarms. It is pretty obvious to all of us that we can't go it alone.

Social Wellness and Your Health

You're probably thinking this sounds pretty dramatic. After all, does it really make a difference if we have a vast social network, or is this just some kind of psychological happy-blabber? I hate to tell you, but there is ample proof that social wellness can affect the *quality* and *quantity* of your life. Based on a *preponderance of the evidence* (my legal term of the day), people will positively affect their physical and mental beings by maintaining a healthy involvement with others. While this book is not designed to be a handbook on social wellness, you will find several studies below to help substantiate that supposition:

- The health impact of social interaction on the residents of Roseto, Pennsylvania was studied in the 1960s. The town was populated primarily by Italian immigrants from the area of Roseto, Italy (yes, they named the new town after their home). In the 1960s, some medical folks noticed that the rate of heart disease in this community was barely half that of the national average. Not only was the data on the lower heart disease a surprise, but *how* it was accomplished was equally astounding. It seems the Roseto residents achieved their heart health *in spite of* breaking all the "heart rules" of the day. The men worked long hours in local slate mines, being constantly exposed to questionable air quality (to say the least). They ate all the "wrong" things, including sausage, pepperoni, salami, ham, cheese, and eggs. They fried food in lard ... and smoked cigars and cigarettes. They drank large amounts of wine. Essentially, according to physicians of the day, they were doing everything backwards!

Medical professionals began to study the Roseto residents, trying to identify a cause for this very positive anomaly. Many factors were considered, such as water supplies and the quality of available medical care, but were all soon ruled out. Inevitably, the study found that it was the *social interdependence of the citizens* that was the reason for the health anomaly. The fact they had maintained their patriarchal system from Italy, complete with its strong social and family ties, was credited with their good health. This social phenomenon actually came to be called the *Roseto Effect* (Egolf, Lasker, Wolf, and Potvin, 1992). Oh, and just in case this doesn't sound very plausible to you, I'll hit you with one more fact. A follow up study during the 1980s found that as ensuing Roseto generations became educated and moved away from the support and interaction of the community, their subsequent mortality rates would soon decline to reflect the rest of society.

- A study by Brigham Young University (Hadfield, 2010) found that social interaction would elevate our survival odds by fifty percent. They noted that a lack of social wellness is worse than not exercising, and twice as bad as being obese. In addition, findings indicated that low social contact was actually as bad as being an alcoholic or equivalent to smoking fifteen cigarettes a day!

- The Grant Study is a well known, seventy five year longitudinal look at a group of Harvard University students. There were a number of valid results, but it became clear that social kinship was a determining factor in how the subjects adjusted throughout their lives. According to George Vaillant (2009) the most important way to sum up those results is to say that "our relationships with other people matter, and matter more than anything else in the world." Not a lot of gray area there.

There are countless other studies that also correlate lack of social health to medical problems and reduced longevity. They include proof that low social wellness can cause a number of things, including a weakened immune system, depression, chronic stress, higher cholesterol levels, double the rate of Alzheimer's disease, and increases in blood pressure, cancer, and heart disease. As stated, our format here is not the place to detail all of these, but rest assured that the bulk of the evidence is so dramatic that it can leave little doubt that social wellness should be a goal of everyone who values their health.

So What Happened to Us?

I believe that anyone over the age of 35 knows that there used to be socialization ... no, really, people were social! Where has the widespread socialization that was so common in the past disappeared to? I surmise that the apex of social interaction was probably from the 1950s into the 1960s. During those post World War II years, nearly everyone was a member of one or more organizations. Fraternal groups, clubs, and civic organizations were all bursting at the seams with members, and were found in every town. These organizations typically functioned to give back to their communities, and served to support their locality in a variety of ways, including monetarily and with volunteer hours. However, the members also received secondary benefits from the social relationships that arose from meetings, barbecues, functions, etc.

Another big social interaction generator was religion. Most families attended the religious service of their choice, and became exposed to the social aspect of the gatherings as well. Of course, even apart from club membership or religious attendance, there were the neighborhood events, such as holiday parties, backyard barbeques and cookouts, card nights, board games, etc. In short ... people talked to people!

As time has passed, many of the civic and fraternal groups have begun a sort of death spiral ... membership has dwindled, members are getting older, and departed members are not being replaced. In fact, according to the book "Bowling Alone" by Robert Putnam (2000), attendance at club meetings is down 58% over the last 25 years. This has caused many groups to close, or operate with greatly reduced numbers. In addition to a reduction in civic group membership, those participating in religious activities has also been on a long slide. Along with the spiritual malaise that results from the ebb of religious involvement, the social reinforcement is also lessened. Make no mistake, this tie between religion and social wellness is very strong ... even as late as 2000, it was noted that nearly half of all memberships in associations and half of all personal philanthropy was generated from a religious background, while half of all volunteering occurred in a religious context (Putnam, 2000). As time progresses, this decreasing church attendance (and loss of associated social involvement) will no doubt have an effect on social wellness as well. As for many organizations, the future looks very grim. The sad part of this trend is two-fold. First, the communities will not be the benefactors of the many good works done by these groups. More important for our format, there will be a significant loss in fraternalism and socialization as well.

What caused this paradigm shift? Numerous theories abound regarding the change. First, we can all agree that along with death and taxes, change is one of the only constants ... so the change in habits should not have been a total surprise. However, despite the theory that change is inevitable, another big mover in the reduction of social relationships has been the deterioration of the traditional nuclear family unit. In the past, it was common for several generations of a family to live together ... if not together, within a short distance of each other. This proximity was a self-generator of interaction, since families met for a variety of activities including meals, parties, holidays, etc. Yet, as people moved away from their family circle for better opportunities, families were often separated by hundreds or even thousands of miles. So, the result was that now the familiar social interaction also fell by the wayside. There can be no argument that the increased societal mobility has impacted social wellness.

Digging a little deeper, a case could be made that the appearance of television was also a big mover with regards to the social shift. Television served as a pseudo-social substitute, and it became easier to get your interaction with the outside world through the tube. Please make no mistake ... the appearance of the television, as well the rapidity of its spread among consumers, has been amazing. For instance, Putnam (2000) notes that in 1950 less than ten percent of homes had a television, while less than a decade later (in 1959) the number of homes with televisions was ninety percent! The long term impact? In 1995, television accounted for 40 percent of the average American's free time (Putnam, 2000). That is pretty dramatic. Unfortunately for us, the rise of television ownership caused more meals in front of the television, limiting inter-familial interaction as well. (In a related but equally unfortunate twist, another byproduct of the television era was the invention of that amazing tin plate loaded with calories, fat, sodium, and carbohydrates ... that popular platter of goodness, the ubiquitous T.V. Dinner! Yuck.) As television became common, we soon found that each room in our homes had to have its own set, serving to further isolate Junior and Sis from Mom and Dad. To illustrate, by the 1990s, over three quarters of all U.S. homes had more than one television. It seems that the impact of television on social wellness can be summed up with two facts. First, on a micro level, surveys show husband and wives spent 3 to 4 times more time watching television than talking (Putnam, 2000). Additionally, Putnam also quantifies the macro toll of the television habit ... each additional hour of watching television correlates to about a 10 percent reduction in civic involvement. So it seems television became a surrogate nanny that serves to provide our social interaction.

We generally came to understand that this new "boob tube" scenario was pretty bad, and came to the realization how impactful this might be on society ... until computers and the internet burst onto the scene! In fact, mimicking the rise in television ownership, 2013 numbers show that 83.8 percent of U.S. households reported computer ownership (File and Ryan, 2014). With the evolution of computer technology, people could live entire fantasy existences in their home, preferring to replace human social interaction with a life lived through their computers.

They can chat ... order food ... do all their shopping ... watch sports ... take classes ... and any number of other things ... while never actually having to communicate personally with another human.

Oh boy ... we were certain that this shadowy cyber world was about as bad as it could get. That is, until we found that technology could combine our mobile telephone with our computers and produce ... the smart phone! It has become blatantly clear that every person on the planet HAS to have a smart phone! In 2015 it was reported that 68 percent of adults in the U.S. had smart phones, a marked increase over the 35 percent that owned them in 2011 (Anderson, 2015). The phone has now invaded the last few areas of social interaction that we all used to have. One only has to sit down at a restaurant and notice that it is not unusual to see entire tables full of people, regardless of age, all intently staring at their phones ... completely indifferent to all those around them. Do you remember our earlier discussion of wellness guru John Kellogg? If so, you probably recall his premise that everyone should "dismiss work, worries, business cares and annoyances while eating." Wise words, but so often going unheeded today.

I can hear it ... many of you bellowing that all this technology is a fantastic breakthrough in time savings and information transfer ... a real study in progress. While at first glance that theory sounds good, I submit that there is more at stake here. Often referred to as the difference in *high touch* and *low touch*, this self-imposed isolation will have long ranging effects. High touch is characterized by interaction ... in other words, communicating with and talking to others. The traditional class taken in a classroom setting might be considered as high touch, due to the interaction of students with the instructor and with each other. Low touch is exactly as you would imagine, a situation with very little human interface. A great example of low touch might be taking an online computer based class where you never actually meet the instructor or your classmates in person, with all communication being done through devices. The sad, almost depressing fact is that the rise of low touch has, and will, continue to produce more and more social isolation.

Maximizing Your Social Wellness

By now, I have no doubt awakened your need for better social wellness! As you have read this section, you began to think "maybe I should be more concerned with this social stuff." You flash back to your younger days, and remember that "social" wasn't always a good thing. You can recall that if you talked too much in class, teachers would tell your parents that you were being a "little too *social*" ... of course this was nicer than saying little Susie is a blabbermouth! However, now you have a better understanding that you need social interaction for wellness. Since we know that it is important to be social, it becomes obvious that this only happens if we associate with ... other people! These people are found everywhere, and can include friends and family, or even others in your area. Even if you get uncomfortable socially, you *must not lose contact* with the rest of the human race! Depending on your situation it can be hard work ... but in the interest of wellness you must continue to try.

There are a number of ideas for strengthening your social wellness. It is important to understand that you need to work on the bonds between you and other people, as well as those between you and your community. Luckily for you, many things you do to strengthen one aspect will cross over to the other. One of the best is pretty simple ... laugh! Laughter is a universal kinship among people, and it crosses all boundaries. Mark Twain noted that the "human race has only one really effective weapon, and that is laughter." Laughing is purported to have any number of physical benefits, including positive effects on things like tension / stress reduction, blood flow, pain relief, blood sugar levels, immune system function, mood improvement, and countless others. Even more important, since other folks much prefer to be with someone that laughs vs. a miserable curmudgeon, it will also help with your goal to connect with others socially. Laughter and a positive attitude make you much more approachable.

Here's another good one ... try to make a standing date. This "forces" you to have social interaction. My wife and I meet one particular couple every month for dinner. We alternate months selecting the restaurant, with the only rule being that it cannot be a restaurant that we have already been to. We have been doing this for about ten years, only missing a couple of months in that entire time. Some dinners were great, others not so much. In fact we often comment that we should have hired ourselves out years ago as mystery diners! Regardless, we all look forward to our outings, since it gives us time to catch up on events, enjoy some conversation without kids or grandkids ... and hopefully enjoy the food!

As a reminder, let's say it again ... your physical wellness is paramount in everything you do. Therefore, it goes without saying that social wellness can be impacted by physical health as well. Since maintaining a level of physical fitness affects your entire wellness spectrum, a great way to strengthen your social component is by joining a gym or a workout group. You have an opportunity to increase your physical wellness, and at the same time meet new people … the classic win / win situation.

Although we have noted that many fraternal and civic groups are shrinking, that does not mean volunteering is dead. Volunteer in any way that you can. It can be very rewarding personally, as well as rendering critical aid and support to your communities. In addition, you will expand your social connections while you join with others interested in the same charitable ideas. I volunteer for several causes that I think are important, and have found that helping out even a couple of hours several times a year can make a difference.

Everyone likes praise, so don't be afraid to complement others. Try your best to find something nice to say about people you meet during your day. Please be authentic, since people know if you are just blowing smoke! Folks will appreciate a genuine gesture, and will remember your efforts. I eat at restaurants daily, and I *never* fail to tell a server "thanks so much for your help today" as I pay the bill. It really can brighten someone's day … I can't begin to tell you the number of times that statement has caused a server to pause and smile appreciatively in return. Oh, leaving a big tip helps too!

Of course, this is not a comprehensive list. As you can tell, opportunities to increase your interaction socially are endless. Your level of discomfort at trying to increase your social footprint may vary slightly, and generally depends on your level of social isolation. Regardless, learn to accept invitations to functions. Make an effort to go out, particularly when you don't really want to. Work on improving your communication skills. Understand the importance of both *speaking* and *listening* when talking to others. Find groups who share your interests. Keep abreast of news, both locally and nationally so that you can have input in conversations. Make a concerted effort, because both you and your society will benefit.

In summation, as we continue to search for the perfect wellness balance, it is compulsory that we address our need as humans to interact. Despite our innate needs, the fact is that today people have less friends ... umm, and no I'm not talking about your number of Facebook friends! Reports note that the average person today has two friends, a number that has steadily declined for several decades. This is cause for concern, since having four quality friends actually serves to increase your health (Rath, 2006). Not only are friendships declining, but people are increasingly living alone. In fact, the Census Bureau reports that the percentage of single person households grew from 17 percent of total households in 1970 to 27 percent in 2012 (Trowbridge, 2013). To make matters even worse, this is only an average, since the number is significantly higher in rural areas. It appears that at the very same time we are starting to fully recognize the criticality of social well being, we are finding ourselves with less friends and more alone than ever. These facts should jolt us to reality.

Like the other five facets of our wellness pie, social wellness is not an "either / or proposition", since you will constantly be at various places along the wellness continuum. You must understand that the search will never be finished, since the quest is a dynamic process. Yet, by strengthening your social component, you will be more positive in everything you do, which will manifest itself both physically and mentally.

Personally ...

As wellness begins to reappear on the radar of many medical practitioners, we have seen an increased awareness that many of their patient's issues may be caused, or at least greatly affected, by social disconnection. Unfortunately, many doctors are either not properly trained to diagnose these problems, or are not willing to step outside of the traditional scientific method theory. An acquaintance of mine (who also happens to be a wonderful doctor) told me that while she does spend much of her time examining her patients and prescribing medicines for their various maladies, she also has seen the value in reminding / informing patients of the need for social interaction as part of their wellness "prescription." Good for you, Doctor Donna.

Physical Wellness

"Lack of activity destroys the good condition of every human being, while movement and methodical physical exercise save it and preserve it."
Plato (Greek philosopher)

I intentionally left this final piece of the wellness pie ... physical wellness ... until the end. I wanted the reader to absorb the importance of physical wellness to all the other pieces of the pie ... and in turn, to overall wellness. If you have read this far, you no doubt have some understanding of the interplay between the various pieces of our wellness pie ... more specifically, you have seen that physical wellness is woven conspicuously throughout each of the other parts of overall wellness.

Let's get down to business ... we only have one body, and while some of the parts can be removed, repaired, or replaced, we are pretty much stuck with our equipment from cradle to grave ... from womb to tomb ... from sperm to worm ... okay, you get the point. We expect our bodies to perform for us when we ask them to work or play. To give your body a chance to produce at its peak, you must prioritize by taking care of the body, and by doing so, reducing your chance of sickness and injury. As our wellness pie suggests, not caring for the physical body may be okay for awhile, but not forever. In short, we need to consider physical wellness.

What the heck is physical wellness? Is it the same as

physical fitness? Good questions. As a society, we began to think about "fitness" somewhere around the 1950s when it was documented that people's inactivity was a major contributor to heart disease. So, in came the fitness programs. For many of us, the term physical fitness conjures up the old school P.E. classes from days gone by … complete with uniforms … coaches … stinky locker rooms … and showering with the rest of your classmates! Putting those wonderful mental images behind … physical fitness generally refers to our body's strength, shape, and cardiovascular abilities … on more generic terms, it refers to the ability of the body to do work. However, fitness programs (then and now) were usually designed to address only the lack of physical activity, and didn't really attempt to address comprehensive *wellness*. Recalling our quest for overall balance, it should be understood that physical fitness is only a part of the wellness aggregate. How about if we say this ... physical fitness contributes to your physical wellness … which in turn contributes to your overall wellness. So for our purposes in this section, we will concentrate on achieving physical wellness as opposed to simply physical fitness.

There is no doubt that physical wellness is more than just fitness. There are many people (and I know a bunch of them) that have the "body beautiful", and are very capable of running, jumping, pulling, stretching, bouncing, hopping, pushing, squatting, lunging, and lifting ... yet they aren't *well*. They lead lives that stress fitness, but are not balanced in other areas of their lives. They should continue to embrace their fitness goals, but also understand that that they should not neglect the other aspects of their being. Keeping with that theory, I feel that physical wellness can be defined as the result of *a proactive balance between physical activity, proper nutrition, and effective health care.* Note in this definition that I begin with the term *proactive*. This is meant to remind you once again that you need to be an *active participant* in your journey toward wellness.

Physical Activity

As the years have passed, there is no doubt that most of us don't work as hard physically as we used to. We don't have to stalk and chase our food ... we don't chop down trees and fashion logs to build our houses ... we don't walk miles to get from place to place ... we don't pick up big rocks to clear our fields. We now have a multitude of labor saving devices that enable us to easily and efficiently do most jobs. Of course, while these devices have made our lives physically easier, they have also taken away much of the built-in activity that used to be a part of our daily lives. But all is not lost ... to receive the missing physical benefits, you just have to replace the activity you aren't currently doing with ... other activities!

Although we examined physical activity in more depth in the Workout chapter, suffice to say that increasing physical activity is at the root of physical wellness. The Center for Disease Control recommends that for a minimum level of fitness, you should perform thirty minutes of moderate intensity aerobic activity most days of the week, as well as do some form of muscle strengthening at least twice a week. If you can't handle the daily thirty minutes of aerobic activity all at once, break it up into two 15 minute sessions or three 10 minute sessions. As a reminder, we showed you how to calculate your aerobic work level by using your heartbeat ... or you can just remember that moderate intensity means that you may break a light sweat and that you will still be able to talk normally while performing the activity.

To reach a minimum strength goal, at least two days a week you should undertake some sort of resistance training. You can work out with resistance bands, use the body weight for resistance (push ups, sit ups, etc.), or lift free weights. Yoga and tai chi also have strength benefits in addition to increasing flexibility. If you aren't sure what to do, go on the internet, ask someone, or hire a trainer. Regardless, don't over-think the whole thing … just use the major muscle groups to push and pull. Again, more information can be found in Chapter 7 of this book. To repeat, at the risk of minimizing the whole deal, the body broken down into its simplest functions is designed to push and pull. If you perform a workout with this in mind, you will be fine.

Okay, these are your basic, minimum guidelines for physical activity. This is a perfect spot to revisit what a regular program that includes aerobic activity and strength exercises can do for you. A workout regimen helps you to control your body weight … reduces the odds of you suffering cardiovascular disease … lowers the odds of strokes … minimizes type 2 diabetes … and combats a number of types of cancer. Workouts increase muscle strength … bone density … stability and balance … while improving your sleep and mental health. Lastly, there is evidence that shows that shows activity increases your life span (Physical Activity and Health, 2015). Research shows people who are physically active for about 7 hours a week have a *40 percent lower risk of dying early* than those who are active for less than 30 minutes a week. Wow, if there was a pill that would do all this for us, we would all race to the pharmacy to get it!

Some more news here ... much of physical wellness is about the choices you make. Staying with the wellness theme, increasing physical activity almost always increases the quality of your life, since being healthy allows you to function at a higher level and maintain your self-sufficiency. Even better news ... the benefits of physical activity are available to everyone, regardless of age, size, sex, or previous experience. Increasing physical wellness doesn't need to involve rocks or logs or hunting game, but it does involve you being active ... at least more than walking from the couch to the refrigerator! Small changes equal big results, especially over time. It is noteworthy that your goal of wellness is meant to be a lifelong journey, so incremental changes added together can make huge impact. When it comes to increasing your physical wellness, famous sportswear manufacturer Nike had it right in their slogan that said ... *Just Do It!*

Proper Nutrition

With respect to nutrition, it's really easy to make the comparison between your body and an automobile. Let's face it, if you neglect the maintenance schedule of your vehicle and fill it with substandard fluids and parts, it is only a matter of time until it leaves you on the side of the road. Understand that your body operates on the same principle ... and when it comes to fueling the body it is absolutely true that the adage "garbage in, garbage out" is valid.

Because of our book's target audience (the overweight and obese), as well as our premise that reducing carbohydrates is the immediate and long term answer, our nutrition suggestions will look slightly different than others you may have seen. For instance, we aren't very interested in having you eat lots of fruit and drink fruit juices. The body treats these things as though you were eating spoonfuls of sugar, causing insulin spikes and resulting in hunger pangs. So we pay much more attention to the glycemic index of food, which is basically how foods affect blood glucose levels. It is far preferable that you eat lower glycemic (low carb) foods, since they digest slower and eliminate the swings in glucose and insulin response.

While this topic is covered in more depth in the *Weight Loss* section (Chapter 4), suffice to say that although we recommend reduced carbohydrate eating, nutrition is paramount. To lose weight and keep it off, you have to eat! The trick is to eat the proper things. Eating reduced carbohydrate foods will result in your feeling full longer. So enjoy your meals, and if you're hungry in between, have some carbohydrate friendly snacks. Endeavor to include protein, as well as grains and low carbohydrate vegetables. Avoid sugar like it is a poison. If you don't take them now, consider adding vitamin and mineral supplements.

Effective Healthcare

I have told you several times in this book about the importance of forging a working relationship with a physician. I'm not going to say that again. I lied ... GO TO THE DOCTOR! I hope you get the idea that it is non-negotiable! Look, nobody can see what is happening inside their body. Find a primary care doctor that you are comfortable with. Your primary care doc isn't the only medical professional that you should see over your life ... of course you shouldn't neglect your teeth, eyes, skin, etc. However, your primary care pro should be at the center of your wellness plan. They will give you a physical, checking your body inside and out. They will have you go to a lab and get some blood work done, and maybe even have you pee in a cup for analysis. They will review the results with you, and suggest ideas to bring your body to a healthier state. After an office visit or two, you and your physician will know the normal readings for things like your weight, blood pressure, cholesterol, and blood sugar levels. Your doc will prioritize your conditions, knowing which problems are the most serious and should be addressed first. Most likely they will prescribe medications if needed, but will also talk about lifestyle changes. They will likely be happy that you are attacking your weight issue by a reduced carbohydrate eating plan. They can also help with any other problems you have, such as alcohol or smoking or sleep problems ... but you have to TELL THEM. To sum it all up, you and your doc should work together as a team, with the common goal of improving your health status. Working in tandem with your physician, you can take responsibility for improving your physical wellness, and in turn your overall wellness.

In a perfect world, you will come across a doctor that is interested in promoting overall wellness, and also agrees with (or at least understands) reduced carbohydrate eating. I feel blessed that for many years, I have been able to establish an association with primary care physicians that fit the bill perfectly. They understand the importance of the working relationship that all parts of the body have with the others. Please don't be shy about going to a physician due to your size, since I promise you that you won't be the first obese person that they have seen (remember that over 65% of the population is overweight, and 35% is obese!). Also, please ... please ... please be honest with your doc. Don't put them (and your health) at a disadvantage by not telling the truth. I promise they aren't going to put all your information on the front page of the newspaper!

Finally, don't resist going to your doctor because you are afraid of what they will find. Their exams and tests may find you are fine, or they may identify some problems. Realize this ... the biggest advances in medicine in our lifetime have been the ability to diagnose any number of maladies at a much earlier stage. Of course, this early detection also permits earlier treatment ... and vastly increased success rates. One thing is for certain, if you choose not to go to the doctor, you'll never be diagnosed with any medical problems. If that's your choice, then you have to remember the following statement: *When you're dumb, you suffer.* Grow up ... go see a doctor.

Oh, and One More Thing

This is a good time to address drinking and sleeping ... but not necessarily together! I'm talking about the need for liquid refreshment and rest ... primarily the body's need for water and sleep.

Most folks generally operate in a partially dehydrated state on a daily basis. Since the body is comprised of at least 60% water, not drinking enough liquids puts the body at a disadvantage. Everyone knows that we should drink more water, but you may not know that although a person can survive for weeks without food, the same person can only make it for about 3 or 4 days without water, depending on the circumstances. Water is an essential part of all processes in the body. It helps to make your blood and saliva, regulates body temperature, is involved in heart rate and blood pressure, removes waste and allows effective digestion. It also lubricates your joints and transports minerals and nutrients throughout the body. That is enough for now, but be assured that water is extremely important to the proper functioning of the machine we call our body.

Hopefully we have agreed on the importance of water to your health, and now you want to know how much water you should drink in a day. Much of the conventional wisdom says that an adult should drink about a half gallon a day. Personally, I feel that number should be adjusted much like medicine dosages ... base it on age, weight, etc. Regardless, I have a fantastic, totally scientific method to tell how you are doing with your water intake ... just take a look at your pee! Seriously, when you urinate, look in the toilet ... if you are hydrated, your urine should be clear or slightly a pale yellow or wheat colored, and have almost no smell. Conversely, if you need more water in your system, your urine will be darker in color and have more smell to it. Now there's a conversation for your next meal time! So, while the color of urine can be affected by some medicines and supplements, as well as by some medical issues, generally if you are drinking enough water your urine should be fairly clear.

Much like the information regarding water intake, there has been an abundance of research regarding the amount of sleep each person needs. The best way to sum up the majority of theories is to say that most folks older than 18 need about 8 hours a night. To no one's surprise, there is no shortage of opinions on the subject, and I have mine also ... lucky for you. Here comes another mind boggling chunk of info ... you need to get ... the amount of sleep ... that allows you to ... feel good the next day! Yep, another epiphany from me to you! Look, there are no "right" amounts of sleep. Your needs are part hereditary, part genetic imprint. It varies daily, and is affected by a myriad of influences (alcohol, caffeine, stress, how deep your sleep is, etc.). The biggest thing to remember is that sleep is how your machine rests, heals, and repairs itself ... so it is vital. Following the common thread of our book, you can function with less than optimal sleep for awhile, but you cannot do it forever ... you will be out of balance. Your physical wellness will suffer and of course this will eventually manifest itself in your overall wellness as well.

While there are no fool proof methods for adequate sleep, there are some constants that work for many people. Make it a habit to get the daily exercise that we have mentioned, since exercise has the byproduct of fatiguing your body. At night, you should also try to maintain a constant schedule. Try to relax for about an hour before hitting the sack ... maybe take a hot bath ... watch a little television or do some reading. Make sure the bedroom is quiet and dark. Room temperature is also important, since most people sleep better when the room is cooler. If your mattress and pillow aren't comfortable, you could be sabotaging yourself before you get started.

Regarding work and sleep, somewhere around 33 percent of all workers work some kind of non - traditional shift (in other words, outside the Monday to Friday, 9 - 5 schedule). Sleep problems for shift workers are fairly common. I worked a rotating shift schedule for over 15 years, including 8 and 12 hour shifts, afternoons and midnights, and weekends as well. After I changed jobs to a straight day shift spot, I designed and taught a *"Coping With Shiftwork"* class to the new shift workers in our company. I assure you, it was called "coping" because *coping is the best you will ever do* ... otherwise it would have been called *"Kicking the Crap Out Of Shift Work!"* The biggest thing I noticed through the years is that many of those who were new to shift work refused to understand that this was a whole new animal. They would work all night, then try to stay awake all day and lead a normal schedule. That might work on occasion ... and most shift workers will tell you they have done it when needed. However, regardless of your reasons, you must get sleep to charge your batteries. Find out what sleep tricks work for you. Ask any shift work veterans that you know for tips ... although shift work is harder on you as you age, shift work veterans have generally found ways to cope. Above all, understand that sleep is not a luxury, it is a necessity.

As we begin to summarize this unit regarding physical wellness, we may want to think of our bodies as medieval castles. It was imperative that castles maintained their structural integrity to ensure no cracks in the walls existed, since cracks made it easy for the enemy to enter. Just like these castles of old, we must strive to protect our bodies ... the best way to do this is by maintaining an overall wellness balance. As a part of this balance, the wellness of our bodies is very important. In this chapter we have made a case for the need to maintain physical wellness, and have suggested that the best plan for your physical well being would consist of a balance between activity, nutrition, and health care. Physical wellness is an important piece of our wellness pie, and is critical for your balance. Recall our earlier definition ... physical wellness is the *proactive balance between physical activity, proper nutrition, and effective health care.* Be proactive … don't wait … get started today.

9   CONCLUSION

Well, it looks like you made it ... the last chapter! I really, really do appreciate you taking time out of your life's schedule to read my book. Along the way, you were exposed to history, math, statistics, biology, anatomy, physiology, economics, legal terminology ... sounds like the first two years of a four year college degree!

The goal of writing this book was for me to become fabulously wealthy, go on extended speaking engagements, and be the guest speaker at numerous motivational seminars. Just in case all that doesn't materialize ... my real goal was to encourage you to take charge of your life through weight loss, workouts, and wellness. My sincere hope is that *at least one person* uses this information to make major changes to their lives ... not because I want any pats on the back, but because I know that this plan works, and would love for it to work for you too. Life is for living ... don't sit around with your lip hanging out and whining about how bad you have it. As noted earlier, changing your way of doing things will be very simple ... but not always easy. If you are overweight or obese, don't wait:

- You've read the book ... make an appointment with your physician tomorrow. Talk to them about eating a reduced carbohydrate diet for the rest of your life, as well as your plan to increase your activity level. Mention that your future goal is a balanced lifestyle, focusing not on disease, but on wellness.

- You've read the *Weight Loss* section … don't delay any longer … commit to start your new way of eating within seven days of reading this book. Research reduced carbohydrate foods … go to the store and buy some … then eat less than 30 net carbs a day. Drink water, and weigh yourself occasionally.

- You've read the *Workout* section … wait 1-2 weeks after you start the new eating plan, then make decisions about whether you are going to work out at home or in a gym. Refer to the book and begin a safe, moderate intensity aerobic exercise plan for 1-2 weeks. After 1-2 weeks, begin your resistance training.

- You've read the *Wellness* section … you know that our pie is cut into six pieces … to achieve maximum wellness the 6 pieces must be balanced. Refer to the book to remind you of the need to balance _within_ each piece of pie, as well as _between_ each piece of pie. This is not a quick trip, it is more of a life-long journey.

Since you may not know me personally, you should understand that I'm pretty much the same as my writing style … I don't take too much very seriously … I'm a little irreverent … I'm fairly straightforward … I'm not real tolerant of folks who are full of excuses … you know, the ones who whine and complain, but don't do anything about it. The most important thing for you to understand is that I _know_ that what I wrote here _works_. It worked for me, and will continue to enrich the rest of my days. If you follow the guidelines in this book, you will lose weight, be better physically, and achieve a much more balanced life. Please follow this plan … you deserve to feel better. Like the title says … it's just that simple.

References

Anderson, Monica. (2015). Technology Device Ownership: 2015. Pew Research Center, Washington, D.C. (October 29, 2015). Retrieved February 13, 2016, from http://www. pewinternet.org/2015/10/29/technology-device-ownership-2015/

Ardell, Donald B. (2000, October). Wellness: Basic definitions of wellness. Retrieved November 26, 2016, from http://www. seekwellness.com/wellness/what_is_wellness.htm

Boyd, Robynne. (2008, February 7). Do People Only Use 10 Percent of Their Brains? Retrieved April 5, 2016, from http://www.scientificamerican.com/article/do-people-only-use-10-percent-of-their-brains/

Carr, Dawn C. (2014, May 5). Use It or Lose It! Retrieved April 5, 2016, from https://www.psychologytoday.com/blog/the-third-age/201405/use-it-or-lose-it

Chiropractic Antitrust Suit Wilk, et al., v. AMA, et al. Index of /08Legal/AT. (n.d.). Retrieved November 11, 2015, from http://www. chirobase.org/08Legal/AT/at034a1.html

Complementary and Alternative Medicine: What People Aged 50

and Older Discuss With Their Health Care Providers.
(2011). Retrieved November 11, 2015, from
https://nccih.nih.gov/research/statistics/2010

Do biomedical models of illness make for good healthcare
systems? (2004, December 9). Retrieved October 29, 2015,
from http://www.bmj.com/content/329/7479/1398

Draper, Dave. (2001). *Brother iron sister steel: A bodybuilder's book.*
[Kindle Version]. Retrieved from www.amazon.com

Egolf, B., Lasker, J., Wolf S., and Potvin, L. (1992). The Roseto
effect: a 50-year comparison of mortality rates. *American
Journal of Public Health,* August 1992: Vol. 82, No. 8, pp.
1089-1092. doi: 10.2105/AJPH.82.8.1089

Employee Tenure Summary. (2014). Retrieved February 12, 2016,
from http://www.bls.gov./news.release/tenure.nr0.htm

Engel, George L. (1977, April 8). The Need for a New
Medical Model: A Challenge for Biomedicine.
Science, Vol 196 (4286), pp 129-136.

File, Thom and Ryan, Camille. "Computer and Internet Use in the
United States: 2013." American Community Survey

Reports, ACS-28, U.S. Census Bureau, Washington, DC, 2014.

Hadfield, Joe. (2010, July 26). Stayin' alive: That's what friends are for. Retrieved December 11, 2015, from https://news.byu. edu/news/stayin'-alive-that's-what-friends-are

Health, United States, 2015 - Individual Charts and Tables: Spreadsheet, PDF, and PowerPoint files. (2016). Retrieved August 27, 2016, from http://www.cdc.gov/nchs/hus /contents2015. htm#015

Helmuth, Laura. (2011, May 19). Top Ten Myths About the Brain. Retrieved March 8, 2016, from http://www. smithsonianmag.com/science-nature/top-ten-myths-about-the-brain-178357288/?no-ist

Hettler, B. 1984. Wellness: Encouraging a lifetime pursuit of excellence. *Health Values: Achieving High-Level Wellness*, 8(4): 13–17.

IHRSA - Newsroom - Health Club Industry Serves 64 Million Americans, an All-time High. (2016, March 8). Retrieved April 12, 2016, from http://www.ihrsa.org/news /2016/3/8/health-club- industry-serves-64-million-americans-an-all-time.html

John, Dan. (2015, May 15). 5 fitness terms that need to die. Retrieved April 24, 2016, from https://www.t-nation. com/opinion/5-fitness-terms-that-need-to-die

Khan, Kasim. (2015). 6 Fundamental Differences Between Religion & Spirituality. Retrieved September 1, 2016, from http://thespiritscience.net/2015/06/07/6-fundamental- differences-between-religion-spirituality/

Koenig, H. G. (2012). Religion, Spirituality, and Health: The Research and Clinical Implications. Retrieved January 16, 2016, from http://www.ncbi.nlm.nih. gov/ pmc/articles/PMC3671693/

Martin, James. (2012, November 6). Spiritual and Religious: The Benefits of Being Both. Retrieved January 16, 2016, from http://www.thinkingfaith. org/articles/20121116_1.htm

McGraw, Philip C. (2003). *The ultimate weight solution: The 7 keys to weight loss freedom.* New York: Free Press

Mercadante, Linda. (2014, February 22). Good news about the 'spiritual but not religious'. Retrieved January 16, 2016, from http://religion.blogs.cnn.com/2014/02/22/good-news-about-the-spiritual-but-not-religious/

Monroe, Mary. (2006, September 1). What Is Wellness? Retrieved December 1, 2015, from https://www.ideafit.com/fitness-library/what-wellness-0

Multiple sclerosis. (2015). Retrieved April 3, 2016, from http://www.mayoclinic.org/diseases-conditions/multiple-sclerosis/symptoms-causes/dxc-20131884

New survey finds Americans care about brain health, but misperceptions abound. (2013, September 25). Retrieved August 28, 2016, from https://www.michaeljfox.org/foundation/publication-detail.html?id=484

"Nones" on the Rise. Pew Research Center, Washington, D.C. (October 9, 2012). Retrieved April 3, 2016, from http://www.pewforum.org/2012/10/09/nones-on-the-rise/

Parkinson's Disease. (June, 2016). Retrieved April 3, 2016, from http://nihseniorhealth.gov/parkinsonsdisease/whatisparkinsonsdisease/01.html

Physical Activity and Health. (2015). Retrieved August 27, 2016, from http://www.cdc.gov/physicalactivity/basics/pa-health/index.htm

Psychology Today. (n.d.). Retrieved April 3, 2016, from https://www.psychologytoday.com/basics/resilience

Puchalski, C. M. (2001). The role of spirituality in health care. Retrieved February 16, 2016, from http://www.ncbi.nlm.nih.gov/pmc/articles/PMC1305900/role of spirituality

Putnam, Robert D. (2000). *Bowling alone: The collapse and revival of American community.* New York : Simon & Schuster

Rasmus, Tara. (2013, May 29). Spirituality Wellness - Does Religion Make You Happy. Retrieved February 16, 2016, from http://www.refinery29.com/spirituality-health

Rath, Tom. (2006). *Vital friends: The people you can't afford to live without.* New York: Gallup Press.

Spirituality May Help People Live Longer. (n.d.). Retrieved February 16, 2016, from http://www.webmd.com/balance/features/spirituality-may-help-people-live-longer

Steinfels, P. (1993). Conversations/Wade Clark Roof; Charting the Currents of Belief For the Generation That Rebelled. Retrieved December 20, 2015, from http://www.nytimes.com/1993/05/30/ weekinreview/conversations-wade-clark-roof-charting-currents-belief-for-generation-that.html

Stephenson, Eric. (2016). The Dalai Lama on Religion and Spirituality. Retrieved September 1, 2016, from http://www.usrepresented.com/2016/03/23/dalai-lama/

Strawbridge WJ, Cohen RD, Shema SJ, Kaplan GA. Frequent attendance at religious services and mortality over 28 years. Retrieved December 23, 2015 from http://www. ncbi.nlm.nih.gov/pmc/articles/PMC1380930/

The Simple Life in a Nutshell ("Biologic Living"). (n.d.). Retrieved November 18, 2015, from http://lifestyle laboratory.com/articles/simple-life-nutshell.html

The Use of Complementary and Alternative Medicine in the United States. (2008). Retrieved November 18, 2015, from https://nccih.nih.gov/research/statistics/2007/ camsurvey_fs1.htm

Trueman, C. N. Medicine in Ancient Rome - History
Learning Site. (2015, Mar 16). Retrieved December 1, 2015,
from http://www. historylearningsite.co.uk/ancient-rome/
medicine-in-ancient-rome/

Trowbridge, Alexander. (2013, August 29). Living alone? You're
not the only one. Retrieved December 21, 2015, from
http://www.cbsnews.com/news/living-alone-youre-not-
the-only-one/

U.S. Department of Health and Human Services. (2009). *Costs of
Complementary and Alternative Medicine (CAM) and
Frequency of Visits to CAM Practitioners: United States, 2007*
(DHHS Publication No. (PHS) 2009–1250 CS204734-C
T34740 (07/2009). Retrieved November 9, 2015, from
https://www.cdc.gov/nchs/data/nhsr/nhsr018.pdf

Vaillant, George. (2009, July 16). "Yes, I Stand by My Words,
'Happiness Equals Love-Full Stop'." Retrieved December
21, 2015, from http://positivepsychologynews.com/
news/george-vaillant/200907163163

Wellness is an active process. (2016). Retrieved July 5, 2015 from
http://www.nationalwellness.org/?page=AboutWellness

What is spirituality? (n.d.). Retrieved August 27, 2016, from

http://au.reachout.com/what-is-spirituality

WHO definition of Health. (n.d.). Retrieved December 2, 2015,

from http://www.who.int/about/definition/en/print.html

Wolpe, Rabbi David. (2013, March 21). *Viewpoint:The
Limitations of Being 'Spiritual but Not Religious."*
Retrieved December 2, 2015, from http://ideas.
time.com/2013/03/21/viewpoint-the-problem-with-being-
spiritual-but-not-religious/

Made in the USA
Lexington, KY
08 September 2018